1990

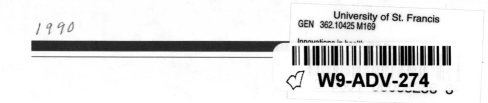
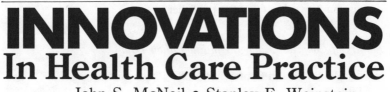

INNOVATIONS
In Health Care Practice

John S. McNeil • Stanley E. Weinstein
Editors

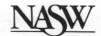

National Association of Social Workers, Inc.
Health/Mental Health Conference

Library of Congress Cataloging-in-Publication Data

Health/Mental Health Conference (1987 : New Orleans,
    La.)
    Innovations in Health care practice.

    Papers from the Health/Mental Health Conference
held in 1987 in New Orleans, sponsored by the National
Association of Social Workers.
    Includes bibliographies.
    1. Community mental health services—Congresses.
2. Community health services—Congresses. 3. Social
service—Congresses. I. McNeil, John S., 1927-
II. Weinstein, Stanley E. III. National Association
of Social Workers. IV. Title. [DNLM: 1. Community
Health Services—congresses. 2. Mental Health
Services—congresses. 3. Social Work—congresses.
W 322 H434i 1987]
RA790.A2H42 1987   362.1'0425   88-31479
ISBN 0-87101-166-2

Printed in the United States of America

Cover and interior design by Vogelsang & Daughters

CONTENTS

FOREWORD

Throughout its history, the National Association of Social Workers (NASW) has placed a high priority on providing continuing education opportunities and on assisting in the integration of the profession. This book represents new strides in both areas.

The NASW conference in 1987 signaled a major shift in the provision of continuing education for social work and it demonstrated NASW's commitment to bringing the profession together. "Social Work '87" was indeed the meeting of the profession, an educational forum that provided knowledge of interest to all social workers in addition to the knowledge presented in the four specialty areas. The format encouraged a new level of integration because participants could move in and out of the four specialty conferences at will. Consequently, they shared ideas with and learned from people who work in other specialties.

In addition to general plenaries, participants met for crosscutting sessions on topics of general interest, such as writing for publication, lobbying, or filing a grievance. They attended informal networking sessions to discuss topical issues, such as licensure, impaired social workers, or peace and justice.

The concept of innovation permeated the conference. Presenters brought the newest in social work knowledge to participants in a variety of formats. They demonstrated videotape training sessions and computer applications. Skills-building workshops, poster sessions, and roundtable discussions augmented traditional presentations. This "conference of conferences" brought 4,500 social workers together for a unique continuing education experience.

By publishing *Innovations in Health Care Practice,* NASW is recording a portion of that continuing education experience for ongoing use by those who attended the conference and others who did not. These articles, which are based on papers presented at the Health/Mental Health Conference, were selected to demonstrate new and expanding areas of practice in health and mental health, as well as efforts to influence policy. We hope that the book will stimulate readers to develop other innovations in practice.

SUZANNE DWORAK-PECK, ACSW
President

MARK G. BATTLE, ACSW
October 1988   *Executive Director*

PREFACE

C hange is a constant in all aspects of our universe. All organisms, however, have the capability of influencing the direction of this change. Adherents of social systems theory inform people that one direction of change is decay and/or extinction (entropy) and the other direction is growth and health (negentropy). This volume is an indication that social work has selected negentropy as its guiding light.

The National Association of Social Workers (NASW), in its decision to hold a professional conference that encompassed four conferences, recognized the need for change to meet the needs of the entire social work profession rather than numerous smaller conferences that separated or departmentalized the profession. This first megaconference or suprasystem conference was held in New Orleans in September 1987. The four specialty groups—(1) health/mental health, (2) family, (3) occupational, and (4) management—met simultaneously, under one umbrella, and attracted more professional social workers than had ever assembled previously. This volume includes articles based on selected papers that were presented at the Health/Mental Health Conference. These articles reflect innovative approaches to dealing with health/mental health problems. These compelling articles also reflect the creativity of social work practitioners and educators and their contributions to the body of professional knowledge. In the articles, the authors examine selected subsystems of consumers, or potential consumers, of social work services. The authors do not simply point out problems but provide guidance on their resolution. Two of the eight articles focus more on policy analysis and the other six are more practice-oriented.

In the first article, "Prospective Payments and Social Work: Obstacles and Opportunities," Terry Mizrahi details and analyzes the major policy and operational issues presented by this piece of legislation. The actions that social workers can take as individuals, collectives, and coalitions to change the system also are emphasized in the article. Audreye E. Johnson in the third article "Health Issues and African-American Women: Surviving But Endangered" depicts this population as having moved beyond facing double jeopardy, but now subjected to triple, quadruple, and quintuple jeopardy because of the history of exclusion of African-American women within American society. Barriers to the acquisition of adequate health care are enumerated and the African-American woman herself and the larger community are exhorted to labor to right this historical wrong.

The second and eighth articles in this volume concern services to mentally ill people, but approach the problem from different perspectives. Laura F. Davis, Agnes B. Hatfield, and Joan P. Bowker address "First-Person Accounts: Lessons for Mental Health Professionals." This absorbing article gives a gripping personalized description of the perceptual and cognitive experiences of the mentally ill person. The authors imply the Indian proverb that one needs to walk a mile in the moccasins of the person before judging that person. Marilyn Kaffie Rosenson, Agnes Marie Kasten, and Mary Elizabeth Kennedy argue the need of "Expanding the Role of Families of the Mentally Ill." They indicate that the role of the family must be expanded on three levels—(1) the nuclear family unit, (2) groups of families similarly affected, and (3) a suprasystem attack on the mental health delivery system.

O. William Farley, Kenneth A. Griffiths, Mark Fraser, and Lou Ann B. Jorgensen enlighten the reader in the article "Rural Social Work: Addressing the Crisis of Rural America." The authors summarize two studies that they had conducted in rural counties. Management strategies are the focus of one study and the process as well as the results of a needs assessment survey are the focus of the other study. Together, the results of the studies provide direction for planning and service delivery in rural areas during times of shrinking resources.

Donald K. Granvold in "Treating Marital Couples in Conflict and Transition" explicates the use of cognitive–behavioral marital therapy for the treatment of this client group. He introduces and explains the underlying theories and language that are essential ingredients of this interventive modality. Material is presented in a lucid manner that can be used readily by the beginning or experienced practitioner. Brenda Wiewel outlines a model for "Healing the Trauma: Treatment for Adult Survivors of Sexual Abuse." Borrowing from the stages of the grief process, she proposes a similar model for the understanding and treatment of adult survivors of sexual abuse. This article is a must reading for all social workers and other therapists who treat this group of clients.

"Chronic Illness and the Quality of Life: The Social Worker's Role," by Shirley A. Conger and Kay D. Moore, explores the impact of chronic illness and disease in the elderly on the patient, the patient's family, and other health care providers. The authors delineate the knowledge needed by the social worker. Additionally, we are reminded of the rapidity with which the size of the elderly population will increase within the next few years.

Innovations in Health Care Practice: Health/Mental Health Conference is a serious attempt to help keep the social work professional abreast of some of the major issues, concerns, and treatment modalities. A book of this type cannot include every problem area. The editors, however, believe the articles included in this volume will prove useful to a majority of social workers.

John S. McNeil, DSW
Stanley E. Weinstein, PhD

PROSPECTIVE PAYMENTS AND SOCIAL WORK:
Obstacles and Opportunities

Terry Mizrahi

The impact of Prospective Payment Systems (PPSs) on the ability of the social work profession to provide quality services at all points along the continuum of care and what can be done to strengthen the role of social workers in present and future health policy are highlighted in this article. It is essential to understand and analyze the policy as well as its implementation, and then identify a variety of strategies and supports needed to improve the health care system, on a long- as well as short-term basis. This includes the identification of some of the initiatives led by or involving social workers already begun at city and state levels and the establishment of an agenda for national action. The following analysis is based on a policy statement developed by the New York City Chapter of the National Association of Social Workers (NASW) in 1987 (New York City Chapter, 1987).

Social workers must end the false dichotomy that either they focus on fixing diagnosis related groups (DRGs) at one end, or work only for a national health service at the other, because both are necessary. But all actions—pragmatic, political, and philosophical—must be taken within the context of a long history of commitment to a progressive health care agenda, most recently articulated in the NASW 1979 *National Health* policy statement (NASW Delegate Assembly, 1979) and reaffirmed as the number one priority by the 1988 Delegate Assembly.

Status of PPS

Social workers are in a unique position, by virtue of their wide range of expertise and responsibilities within the health care profession, to evaluate and influence health care policy. Professional training and practice at all points within the health care delivery system enable social workers to assess the availability and quality of the care offered. Although, as a rule, social workers are not in a position to judge the necessity of specific medical procedures or decisions, their understanding of the complexity of patient needs and the network of services required to meet those needs enables them to evaluate each patient's situation from a broad perspective, provide a range of skilled services, link clients to appropriate community resources where available, and identify problem areas of unmet needs.

This perspective on both the policy and delivery levels places social workers in an excellent position to analyze the effects of PPS and the DRG reimbursement system, in particular, on the quality of patient care. PPS is the model for future health care reimbursement both at the state and federal levels. All-payor systems (including Medicare and private insurance) based on prospective pricing have been initiated in most states, and eventually will cover psychiatric as well as medical care provided within institutional and community-based settings.

PPS was enacted by Congress as part of the Social Security Amendments of 1983. It is considered the most radical change in the history of Medicare. Until 1983 hospitals were reimbursed retrospectively by Medicare for their costs, an action also known as cost-plus reimbursment. Attempts in the 1970s to contain costs through peer review (Professional Standards Review Organizations) and health planning mechanisms (known as regional Health Systems Agencies) were ineffective because there were few sanctions included in these programs. In 1983, prospective pricing was mandated. By basing reimbursement on a fixed rate per case, set prospectively rather than retroactively, PPS has reversed the financial incentives by which Medicare had compensated hospitals for patient services. The rate of reimbursement is based on a system of close to 500 DRGs, categories of illness calculated on the national average of cost per diagnosis. Proposed changes by the Department of Health and Human Services Health Care Financing Administration (HCFA) for fiscal year 1988 include a major expansion of DRG categories covering alcohol and drug abuse.

The explicit philosophy behind PPS is cost containment and the shifting of the responsibility of care for non-acute-care patients to nonhospital settings (Caputi & Heiss, 1984; Kotelchuck, 1984, 1986a). The former reimbursement policy encouraged inefficient use of resources, unnecessary diagnostic and treatment procedures, lengthy hospital stays, in general, erring on the side of overuse or "system abuse." Current PPS/DRG policy, without careful monitoring, encourages the opposite—in general, erring on the side of too little or "system neglect."

PPS Philosophy and Implementation

Beginning research, investigation, and reports offered by patients and health care professionals raise many issues (American Society of Internal Medicine [ASIM], 1988; Kotelchuck, 1986b; Senate Special Committee on Aging, 1985). The implementation of PPS policy has been likened to "psychiatric deinstitutionalization" policy of the past 20 years. For many patients, it has clearly resulted in the curtailment of access to or discharge from hospitals, without an adequate continuing health care system able to meet their needs. But unlike the deinstitutionalized psychiatric patient, many of those discharged as a result of the PPS cost-containment policies are not in the public's eye. They tend to disappear into their own homes (however inadequate) or over-stressed family systems; or they become the burden of long-term health care facilities. In other cases, they return to the acute-care hospital periodically in a more debilitated state than previously. This is known as the "revolving door" syndrome. The more invisible nature of these individuals, combined with the lack of systematic research, allows the myth of success, based on shorter hospital stays and increased hospital profits, to survive (Feder, Hadley, & Zuckerman, 1987; Fitzgerald, Fagan, Tierney, & Dittus, 1987).

Any serious analysis of the effect of PPS on the quality of patient care must start with the concept on which it is predicated, namely, cost containment. Cost containment, while an acceptable goal, should not be pursued at the expense of quality, comprehensive care. By limiting its focus to cutting costs, PPS encourages a mentality that ignores the patient's total health needs. This formal and emphatic injection of marketplace values into the American health care system reflects a retrenchment philosophy that moves in the direction of "back to the alms house." In the past, hospitals have been used to compensate for inadequate community resources and for the general lack of available preventative and rehabilitative services. Reimbursement formulas encouraged the expansion of hospital-based care. More appropriate use of in-patient hospital care now requires that needed services once provided in the hospital be available elsewhere. Paradoxically, at a time of greater need for nonhospital services, cutbacks in

Medicare, Medicaid, home care, and other related services to patients and their families are occurring.

The social work profession has rejected this regressive stance and stands unconditionally opposed to any policy that, directly or indirectly, places the individual's right to adequate health care at odds with a health care provider's legitimate concerns for financial stability. To ensure this, the 1979 NASW Delegate Assembly endorsed, as part of its policy statement on national health, the development of prospective or predetermined schedules of rates of reimbursement. However, it did so within the context of a national health care program that would ensure equal access to the entire population of comprehensive services "which maintain optimal health, prevent illness and disability, ameliorate the effects of unavoidable functional incapacities, and provide supportive long-term and terminal care" (NASW Delegate Assembly, 1980, p. 16.3). The profession must not lose sight of these long-range goals.

Presumably, PPS has targeted inflated medical costs not controlled by a retrospective Medicare reimbursement policy, which offered no incentives for restricting costs. By limiting the reimbursement amount for a specific illness through the use of a DRG formula, it is assumed that the incentives will be for a reduction of unnecessarily long hospital stays and a more efficient use of time and resources. Initial results from acute-care hospitals indicate mixed reviews, depending on the type of hospital and region of the country. In some areas, this has resulted in shorter in-patient stays, a reduction in the use of services and supplies, and increased hospital profits. There is, however, no corresponding evidence of reductions in the needs of patients or in the increased ability of community-based care facilities to fulfill shifting, but continuing, health needs. In fact, patient needs are likely to increase based on demographics alone, and neither state nor federal proposals is adequately addressing the growing need for both home health and long-term institutional care.

Problems with the System

Under PPS, many patients are being discharged in a less-recovered state than previously, commonly referred to as the "quicker and sicker syndrome" (Annas, 1986; California Medical Review, 1987; Fragin, 1986). All health professions are concerned that the present health care system is being strained beyond its capacity, and that alternative care settings are unable to provide the level of service previously provided within acute-care hospitals. A 1986 survey conducted by the Massachusetts Chapter of NASW and the Senate Human Services Committee found that "sixty-four percent of the social workers surveyed had clients so sick upon discharge that they required subsequent rehospitalization, with inappropriate DRGs cited as the cause" (Massachusetts Chapter, 1986). A survey of internists' experiences under DRGs revealed that although DRGs heightened physician consciousness over the cost of care, they also resulted in diminished hospital services, premature discharges, delayed admission of patients and other negative effects (ASIM, 1988).

When the PPS strategy is combined with the situations of many older and poor patients, problems ensue. The health crises of these groups often are characterized by chronic illness, a multiplicity of interacting ailments and impairments, and fluctuating mental impairment that is exacerbated by social and economic factors. The rigid and limited disease-specific DRG formula, based on a primary diagnosis, can be inappropriate and even harmful for many patients, particularly the elderly and the poor (Kotelchuk, 1985). A far broader definition of illness is needed—one that goes beyond a narrow medical assessment and acknowledges the complex interrelationship of social and physical needs of these populations that generally require a longer recovery period or sustained in-home or nursing home care.

What PPS does not consider is that the health care system is a complex network of interdependent services along a continuum of care. The acute-care hospital is but one point along this continuum that includes chronic-care hospitals, rehabilitation centers, nursing homes, hospices, and care based in the home. PPS focuses on this one point and establishes strict medical criteria for acute-care reimbursement, thus restricting access to or continuation of care at this point. The result, therefore, is a shift in responsibility for care to alternate points along the continuum with no corresponding increase in services or financing at these points.

National Medicare PPS policy is made by HCFA and is implemented through statewide and regional peer review organizations (PROs) whose responsibility is basically to monitor cost containment and, secondarily, to monitor quality of care (Kotelchuck, 1987). Pressure from consumer and health advocates has resulted in Congress strengthening the protections safeguarding patients' rights to quality care by establishing an elaborate appeals process for patients denied continuing hospitalization (American Association of Retired Persons, 1985). Currently, hospitals are required to give each Medicare patient a copy of HCFA's Patients' Rights Message and a written notification of denial of services. Some states, such as Massachusetts and New York, have instituted even more elaborate procedures. Unfortunately, many patients and families who are still unaware of their rights and protections find the appeals process confusing, or they do not receive adequate information and interpretation of that information. Attempts to improve and mandate discharge planning are a step in the right direction, but do not always ensure that timely, informed, satisfactory, and realistic plans are professionally implemented by social workers.

Although PPS using DRGs has greatly affected discharge planning by increasing its visibility and importance in the hospital, it also has increased the workload for those trying to cope with the changes (Feather & Nichols, 1986; Pachner & Wattenberg, 1985; Reamer, 1985). Discharge planning under PPS—once the cornerstone of professional hospital social work practice—has greater pressure on it. It now serves patients who are more sick entering and leaving hospitals, in less time, with fewer and often uncoordinated resources inside and outside the hospital. Most social work departments that have retained primary management responsibility for discharge planning have not experienced a reduction in staffing levels or functions ("Survey Shows," 1987). Hence, the importance of social work controlling this essential hospital function cannot be overestimated. However, in many settings, the quality and scope of social work responsibilities have changed under DRGs, resulting in an acknowledged and growing problem of professional staff recruitment and retention. These problems need the urgent, concerted attention of the whole profession and its allies.

Strategic Approaches

Because there are many related health policies and programs that affect the social worker's ability to provide quality patient care, it is difficult to isolate PPS/DRG strategies from related issues concerning, for example, home care, long-term care, and health maintenance organizations (HMOs). However, it is important not to make DRGs an acute-care, in-patient hospital issue alone. Politically and philosophically, strategies should be devised with three goals in mind:

1. Unifying the profession (rather than compartmentalizing or dividing it).

2. Connecting social work and patient issues (rather than separating them or giving greater priority to one).

3. Defining "the patient" universally to include the working and middle class (without losing sight of the special concerns of the medically, economically, and socially needy).

With these three goals in mind, the strategy used must be a multilevel and multipronged one. To be most effective, social workers must focus simultaneously on the larger picture and the specific DRG implementation.

There are three levels on which to work **Levels**
for change: (1) making current DRG policy
work, (2) reforming PPS/DRG policy, and (3) creating a genuine "right
to health care" program. Clearly, at the third level, social workers must
continue to actively promote a national health policy that ensures a right
to comprehensive health care regardless of race, financial status,
ethnicity, religion, age, gender, sexual orientation, or geographic loca-
tion. In joining the National Health Care Campaign and other coalitions,
NASW has already moved in that direction (Harris, 1986). Within this
long-range agenda, social workers should support all legislative thrusts
to increase health resources through Medicaid, Medicare, and new approaches such as the Bradley/Waxman Bill to improve home health
services. However, social workers must continue to educate clients and
the public about the limitations of specific proposals (especially the
Reagan Administration's Catastrophic Health Insurance Proposal) as
well as the limitations of such piecemeal approaches to health reform.

The second level is changing the current DRG system to make
it equitable and to ensure quality health care. Reforms at this level
should be addressed primarily to HCFA and PROs. Several substan-
tive revisions are suggested, as follows:

• Adjustment must be made in the formulation of the DRG
categories so that PROs can assess a broader range of factors that affect the need for and length of stay in hospitals. DRG classifications
should include an indicator for severity of illness, the chronic and in-
teractive nature of multiphysical ailments, particularly among the
elderly and the poor, and social and psychological factors that affect
medical needs such as inadequate housing, homelessness, impaired
mental status, and status of family supports.

• Adjustments must be made in the interpretation by PROs of the
concept of "medically necessary" used in determining the need for
continued hospitalization. This should include social factors that affect medical status such as the patient's readiness to leave and the support and service network in place for the patient. Otherwise, the
"revolving door/multiple admissions" scenario will increase. A progressive step in that direction was taken by the New York State Health
Department in its 1988 insurance regulations for non-Medicare DRG
reimbursement. These regulations stated that patients can be
discharged only if they are "medically" ready and if the necessary
post-hospitalization plans are "reasonably" in place.

• The function of PROs should be expanded further to monitor the
planning for pre- and post-hospital care, as it now includes monitoring the transfer of patients from private to public hospitals. HCFA
needs to mandate investigation by PROs of areas not previously
covered, such as refused hospital admission, emergency room

turnaways, and patient interviews as followup on appeals. PROs should include social workers as reviewers and staff to ensure that the social history and status are part of the medical diagnosis and treatment and, in particular, to promote proper discharge planning and to monitor the efficacy of discharge plans after execution.

• Because discharge or, more appropriately, continuity-of-care planning, is mandated, it must be considered covered by Medicare and receive the appropriate financial resources, guidelines, and support allocated for this important professional function.

• The current patient protection and appeals process needs continued strengthening, simplification, and standardization. The rights messages of HCFA patients should be sent to all social security/Medicare recipients on a regular basis to alert the elderly to the process *before* they require hospitalization. The statement should be made available in several languages to ensure the enforcement and implementation of all patients' rights. The appeals process should be simplified so that it is the same whether the physician agrees or disagrees with a hospital's decision to discharge a patient. There should be no liability to the patient during an appeal.

• HCFA should mandate independently funded patient advocate or ombudsperson systems inside hospitals and/or in the community to assist vulnerable patients and their families and to help monitor hospital and PRO activity. Penalties for deliberate and pervasive violations of patients' rights should be assessed at appropriate levels.

The first level of making change involves improving the current system. This is a delicate situation because social workers must be both interpreters and implementers of the system and also act as advocates for clients and their families. Nevertheless, there are two steps social workers can take while advocating for these improvements and a national health care program.

1. Social workers must work to improve **Interim Steps** the current patient appeals process.
Because of the complexity of the appeals process for denial of hospital admittance or early discharge, it is strongly suggested that patients seek the assistance of a health advocate while proceeding with the appeals process. Because PROs are government contractors mandated to monitor the quality of Medicare services, they implement federal policies and represent professional and provider perspectives. Social workers, with knowledge of the system, can guide and support patients and families throughout the complicated review process. When the hospital social worker is unable to be the patient's primary health advocate, information about independent advocacy programs or hot

lines should be made available to the patient. If there are no such groups in a community, the local NASW chapter may wish to consider facilitating their development.

2. The social work role in educating seniors and senior groups must be addressed. Specific education and information provided by social workers on the DRG system can empower older persons to give educational forums that inform consumers of their rights and benefits. Training and education will enhance the health advocacy stance of seniors on their own individual and collective behalfs. This education should stress the following points:

• Discharge planning is an activity that needs to begin before hospitalization. Many elderly who are scheduled for hospitalization are unaware of the need to plan their post-hospital care well ahead of time. There is a need to educate families and the elderly about the scarcity of community resources and the amount of time it often takes to begin services. There is a need to involve families in assessing and facilitating the appropriate level of their participation.

• Elderly patients need to know that under Medicare they generally are entitled to two free days of hospital stay after receiving a written hospital notice of discharge. To receive these two free days, the patient must appeal the hospital's discharge decision. It is recommended that the patient who feels that he or she is not ready to leave the hospital contact a professional advocate to assist with the appeals process and the confusion and misinformation involved.

Arenas for Action

In this section, some of the programs and approaches taken and suggested by social workers are discussed briefly. Projects take additional energy at a time when the demands on social workers, regardless of level or setting, are increasing. Nevertheless, social workers have the experience, expertise, and knowledge to make a difference, and ultimately to make life better for themselves and their clients (Kerson, 1985; Sosin & Caulum, 1983; Mailick & Rehr, 1981).

There are seven arenas of involvement. Social workers may choose to become involved in any or all of these arenas:

1. *Individual Worker*—Provides information and advocacy services to clients and documents problems anecdotally and statistically from individual caseloads.

2. *Department*—Systematically develops mechanisms for information, referral, and resource coordination, and documents systemic problems for groups of clients.

3. *Agency*—Urges the agency or institution to take public or behind-the-scenes positions or alters their own policies where possible.

4. *Interorganization*—Involves agencies whose functions are coordination, planning, and policy.

5. *Community*—Initiates or participates in networks, alliances, and coalitions.

6. *Professional*—Involves NASW and other more specialized social work organizations, such as the Society of Hospital Social Work Directors (SHSWD) and the Oncology Social Workers' Network.

7. *Political*—Targets the decision makers—those who have influence and authority—for action. At this level, this means involvement in pressure (lobbying) or partisan (electoral) politics.

Decisions on which levels to work should be based on the following criteria:

• the intensity and extensiveness of the problems as viewed and experienced directly by the social worker,

• the existence and effectiveness of local professional and community organizations,

• the access to and responsiveness of influential elected and appointed officials, and

• the skills social workers have to offer.

Whether working directly with clients, community organizations, or public officials, the following four action strategies should be considered:

1. *Education.* This involves educating social workers and their constituencies about the problems and their consequences for clients, the profession, communities, and society. To cite two examples, in late 1986 the New York City Chapter of NASW created a PPS task force that developed a simple form for social workers to document client problems, and in 1986, the Massachusetts Chapter of NASW conducted a survey of hospital social workers. Needless to say, forums should be established to publicize systemic or intense problem situations. Continued public education about the four "R's" under PPS: (1) rights, (2) responsibilities, (3) redress or remedy (when things go wrong), and (4) resources also is needed.

2. *Outreach.* This involves reaching individuals and organizations in the seven arenas identified previously by holding workshops, forums, and conferences and using media (organizational as well as mass media). For example, the New York Chapter of NASW held a conference in 1987 on PPS cosponsored by the New York metropolitan area chapter of SHSWD. At that meeting, Susan Kinoy, a social work advocate, urged social workers to reach out to senior advocacy groups. Her organization, the Villers Foundation (located in Washington, D.C.), and the National Health Care Campaign are resources to identify senior and other health advocacy organizations.

3. *Coalition Building.* This involves encouraging like-minded, concerned organizations to join forces. Although in some agencies and communities there are tensions between social work and other health professions such as nursing and medicine, the time is ripe for all members of the "health care team" to unite (Abramson & Mizrahi, 1986). For example, a coalition of groups in Massachusetts was responsible for successfully getting on the state ballot act, a nonbinding referendum on a national health program that was approved by a two-to-one margin (Danielson & Abrams, 1987). In New York State, NASW, SHSWD, and a patient advocacy coalition known as the DRG Strategy Group have been working to influence the New York State Health Department to strengthen both patient protection and social work roles in the health code.

4. *Advocacy.* This involves persuading gatekeepers and policy makers to implement or improve services that work in the best interest of clients—individually and collectively. The goal of advocacy is to link case advocacy and class advocacy and to acquire skills in both arenas. Social workers need to teach each other the ways in which they successfully negotiate with or on behalf of an individual client, while recognizing that in a time of political and economic conservatism the pool of available resources and services also must be expanded; otherwise one person's gain may be another's loss.

Education, outreach, coalition building, and advocacy should occur on local, state, and national levels (Mahaffey & Hanks, 1982). As reported recently (Harris, 1986; "Experts Panel Examines," 1988) health policy and financing issues are already a priority area for staff and volunteer leadership. This leadership should be commended for this and is encouraged to continue on all fronts.

In addition, social workers can call for the following:

• A national study on the impact of PPS on social work to be conducted by the National Center for Social Policy and Practice.

• Adaptation by the next Delegate Assembly of a major policy statement on PPS. This can be built on the PPS resolution already passed by the 1988 Delegate Assembly.

• Strengthening coalition building efforts toward national health care reform.

• Production of a resource packet with background materials on PPS for local NASW chapter initiatives.

This is a challenging time to be a social worker in the health care field. The rapid and almost revolutionary nature of the fiscal changes in the health care system today require active participation by all social workers. Self-interest and altruism are interwoven inextricably as work toward an equitable and just health system for workers and clients alike is undertaken.

Abramson, J. & Mizrahi, T. (1986). Strategies for enhancing collaboration between social workers and physicians. *Social Work in Health Care, 12,* 1–22.

American Association of Retired Persons. (1985). *Knowing your rights: Medicare's prospective payment system.* Washington, DC: Advocacy Services Project Department.

American Society of Internal Medicine. (1988). *The impact of prospective payment on patient care: A survey of internists experiences under DRGs.* Washington, DC: American Society of Internal Medicine.

Annas, G. J. (1986). Your money or your life: Dumping uninsured patients from hospital emergency wards. *American Journal of Public Health, 76,* 74–77.

California Medical Review, Inc. (1987). *Premature discharge study.*

Caputi, M. A. & Heiss, W. A. (1984). The DRG revolution. *Health and Social Work, 9,* 5–12.

Danielson, D. & Abrams, S. (1987). They did it in Massachusetts: A report on the first national health referendum. *Health PAC Bulletin, 17,* 16–18.

Feather, J. & Nichols, L. O. (1986). Hospital discharge planning for continuity of care: The national perspective. In E. G. Hartigan and D. J. Brown (Eds.), *Discharge planning for continuity of care* (pp. 71–78). New York: National League for Nursing.

Feder, J., Hadley, J., & Zuckerman, S. (1987). How did Medicare's prospective payment system affect hospitals? *New England Journal of Medicine, 317,* 867–872.

Fitzgerald, J., Fagan, L., Tierney, W., & Dittus, R. (1987). Changing patterns of hip fracture care before and after implementation of the prospective payment system. *Journal of the American Medical Association, 258,* 218–221.

Fragin, S. (1986, January 21). Sicker and quicker. *The Village Voice,* pp. 17–19.

Harris, D. (1986). Making the case: Social work and the health care revolution. *NASW News, 31,* 2.

Kerson, T. S. (1985). Responsiveness to need: Social work's impact on health care. *Health and Social Work, 10,* 300–307.

Kotelchuck, R. (1984). Baring costs: How the DRG system works. *Health/PAC Bulletin, 15,* 7–12.

Kotelchuck, R. (1985). Poor diagnosis, poor treatment: How the DRG system affects hospitals that serve the poor. *Health/PAC Bulletin, 16,* 7–13.

Kotelchuck, R. (1986a). In the grip of PPS: How the prospective payment system is transforming hospital care. *Health/PAC Bulletin, 17,* 7–10.

Kotelchuck, R. (1986b). And what about the patients?: Prospective payment's impact on quality of care. *Health/PAC Bulletin, 17,* 3–17.

Kotelchuck, R. (1987). Watchdog on a short chain: How good are PPS's quality-of-care reviewers? *Health/PAC Bulletin, 17,* 19–22.

Mahaffey, M., & Hanks, J. W. (Eds.). (1982). *Practical politics: Social work and political responsibility.* Silver Spring, MD: National Association of Social Workers.

Mailick, M., & Rehr, H. (Eds.). (1981). *In the patient's interest: Access to hospital care.* New York: Prodist.

Massachusetts Chapter, National Association of Social Workers. (1986, December). Effects of DRGs on quality health care: Survey by Massachusetts Chapter, NASW, and Senate Human Services Committee.

National Association of Social Workers Delegate Assembly. (1980). *National Health* (A Policy Statement). Silver Spring, MD: National Association of Social Workers.

New York City Chapter, National Association of Social Workers. (1987). *Prospective payment systems.* Silver Spring, MD: National Association of Social Workers.

Pachner, M. A., & Wattenberg, S. (1985). The impact of DRGs on hospital social service departments. *Social Work, 30,* 259–261.

Reamer, F. G. (1985). Facing up to the challenge of DRGs. *Health and Social Work, 10,* 85–94.

Sosin, M., & Caulum, S. (1983). Advocacy: A conceptualization for social work practice. *Social Work, 28,* 12–17.

Senate Special Committee on Aging. (1985). *Impact of Medicare's prospective payment system on the quality of care received by Medicare beneficiaries.* Washington, DC: U.S. Government Printing Office.

Staff. (1987). Survey shows social work gains in staffing, discharge planning. *Social Work Administration Newsletter* (of the Society for Hospital Social Work Directors of the American Hospital Association), *12,* 1–6.

Staff. (1988). Experts panel examines health care dilemmas. *NASW News, 33,* 10.

FIRST-PERSON ACCOUNTS:
Lessons for Mental Health Professionals

Laura F. Davis, Agnes B. Hatfield, and Joan P. Bowker

F irst-person accounts of people with major mental illnesses speak to mental health professionals by giving an inside view of those illnesses. Knowledge and understanding of clients' experiences is the underpinning for all work in mental health. The deinstitutionalization of former patients makes this more important because these people are now in the community in numbers and in ways that are new to many mental health professionals. Community living demands more daily choices than may be needed in the asylum of an institution. Community-based treatment must be more individualized. The professional needs to recognize that the client is coping with an ever-changing inner world that is without consistency and continuity as well as with the ordinary frustrations of life. First-person accounts can provide a link between the professional and mentally ill people who experience life through their sensory perceptions, physical self, emotions, and intellect, which are mediated at times through the screen of the disease. These first-person accounts offer the mental health professional an inside view of the illness (Hatfield, in press) and practical advice on how to proceed with treatment.

First-person accounts exist in books, in professional journals, in government reports, and on videotape. The authors, by definition victims of mental illness, include nurses, physicians, social workers, and others who can give professionally and personally informed insights. For example, Brundage is a nurse who provides professionally oriented insights. Leete is particularly articulate about her experiences garnered from 20 years of schizophrenia. Her accounts are available on videotape and in two articles. The best scholarly sources of first-person accounts are Freedman (1974) who synthesized over 50 autobiographical books and articles, and the works of Torrey (1983), Anscombe (1987), and Kaplan (1964).

Empathy is a basic ingredient in helping relationships that has taken on many meanings (Gladstein, 1983). The most useful for the professional who will work with those with severe mental illnesses is cognitive empathy or understanding another's thinking or feeling and understanding how the other perceives the world. Current work with persons with chronic mental illness focuses on a combination of treatment methods, including medication, social skills training, and family education. Empathy and rapport are needed to implement the treatments effectively (Hogarty et al., 1986).

The necessity of developing empathy and rapport as the basis of a working relationship with any type of client is familiar to social workers and other mental health professionals. It is the work of the professional to translate technology or methodology into a social reality through the helping relationship. With better understanding of the illness by professionals, the alienation and loneliness of the mentally ill person should be reduced. Strauss (1986) emphasizes the importance of understanding the personal side of schizophrenia in the field of psychiatric rehabilitation. There is growing evidence that the nature of the person as a person is an important part of the course and the outcome of schizophrenia. Leete (1987b) graphically describes the efforts she has made in her own behalf over the more than 20 years of the course of her illness—the efforts to recognize the illness and control it, and to establish and maintain a full sense of her own autonomy and identity. Brundage (1983) recalls her recovery from mental illness and concludes that

> the effectiveness in reaching and working with patients rests largely upon the ability of the caregiver to perceive and comprehend how particular patients are experiencing their illnesses . . . Feedback that is understandable to patients in their world is the essence of helpfulness. (p. 585)

Assistance has two aspects: (1) helping to find a place in the world of meaning and (2) helping to find a place in the world of reality. Professionals now emphasize concrete helping, that is, a place to live, an income, a job, satisfying relationships with family and friends, good medical care, and so on. Whatever the specifics, an empathic relationship can move the work forward and create a better fit between the person and the available resources. Although work with the severely mentally ill person probably will not include therapy as commonly defined, there is an element of the therapeutic relationship in working together toward goals. In addition, the mentally ill may want and benefit from supportive therapy. It may be difficult, however, for the chronically mentally ill person to maintain a therapeutic relationship because of the limitations that the chronically mentally ill person has for establishing reciprocal relationships (Carpenter, 1986). Perseverance on the part of the professional may be rewarding, however. McGrath (1984) tells of the support she felt she received from a mental health professional who seemed to understand her in the grip of the illness:

> In the . . . book I've read, a doctor writes that psychotherapy is useless with schizophrenics. How could he even suggest that without knowing me, the one over here in the corner, who finds a lot of support, understanding, and acceptance with my therapist? Marianne is not afraid to travel with me in my fearful times. She listens when I need to release some of the "poisons" in my mind. She offers advice when I'm having difficulty with just daily living. She sees me as a human being and not only a body to shovel pills into or a cerebral mass in some laboratory. Psychotherapy is important to me, and it does help. (p. 639)

This statement illustrates the importance of individualizing the client's program. Although psychosocial rehabilitation in combination with medication management has become an important form of treatment for schizophrenics, it does not provide a formula that can be uniformly applied to all. Social work historically has expressed concern for the person in the environment. In this case, social workers are called on to be concerned with the task of understanding and helping the person in the illness in the environment. This means not being caught in the cant of a specified form of treatment to the exclusion of other resources that may be useful to the client.

A note of caution is in order, as Kaplan (1964) points out. The patient's account of the experience should not be taken for the experience itself. The experience tends to have qualities difficult for ordinary language to communicate. After describing her experiences of an inanimate object coming to life, Sechehaye (1951) stated, "This was not quite exact, but I did not command the words to express the fear . . . " (p. 59). In addition, there is always some selectivity and distortion and forgetting. There are patients who are not as articulate, whose experience is not shared. Nevertheless, these accounts come from those who know what the outsider can only infer.

The Experience of Mental Illness

Persons with mental illnesses describe experiencing the world through the screen of the illness. Their world is changed in response to illness-induced alterations including altered perceptions, cognitive confusion, changes in emotions, and changes in sense of self. Their inner worlds are unpredictable and often chaotic. The mental health professional is then dealing with a person who may have difficulty carrying out ordinary tasks but who is coping with experiences that would present problems to anyone.

Altered Perceptions

In mental illness, the sensory perceptions may be sharpened or dulled. Sights and sounds may appear more vivid and distinct. The mentally ill person may attempt to make sense of what is heard. The following account gives a sense of how the world appears to one with mental illness:

> During several nights when I could not get to sleep, a recurrent crackling noise in the wall of our bedroom became noticeable at shorter or longer intervals; time and time again it woke me as I was about to go to sleep. Naturally we thought it was a mouse . . . but having heard similar noises innumerable times since then, and still hearing them around me every day in daytime and at night, I came to recognize them as undoubted divine miracles—they are called "interferences" by the voices talking to me. (Schreber, 1955, p. 64)

The mentally ill person may focus on smells: "I smelled blood and decaying matter where no blood or decaying matter could be found (for example in the classrooms at school)" (Bockes, 1985, p. 488). Other aspects of the environment may dominate the attention, as described here: "The colors appear brighter, alluring almost, and my attention is drawn into the shadows, the lights, the intricate patterns of textures the bold outlines of objects around me. It's as if all things have more of an existence than I do . . . everything is a wonder" (McGrath, 1984, p. 639). On the other hand, some people with mental illness report that their senses are dulled, that noises are muffled, or that their vision is dulled (Freedman, 1974).

Attention may become focused on minor details:

> For the greater part of the day I sat in a chair, gazing fixedly before me, or plunged in absorbed contemplation of a tiny spot; a spot

which, no bigger than a grain of pepper, could hold me for an hour without any urge to shift my eyes from their absorption in this microscopic world. Only a strong force could pull me away from it . . . . (Sechehaye, 1951, p. 56)

Torrey (1983) illustrates how the disease interferes with the ability to synthesize information and therefore the ability to engage in conversation:

When people are talking I have to think what the words mean. You see, there is an interval instead of a spontaneous response. I have to think about it and it takes time. I have to pay all my attention to people when they are speaking or I get all mixed up and don't understand them. (p. 15)

Minor (1981) reveals how this type of problem affected her interaction with hospital staff: "The staff members were encouraged to carry on conversation with the patients. A simple question, 'Do you live with your mother?' seemed too hard to answer. Unsuccessfully, I tried to answer . . . " (p. 317).

Routine activities can become difficult tasks, as illustrated in the following example from Torrey (1983):

I can't concentrate on television because I can't watch the screen and listen to what is being said at the same time. I can't seem to take on two things like this at the same time especially when one of them means watching and the other means listening. On the other hand I seem to be always taking in too much at one time and then I can't handle it and can't make sense out of it. (p. 15)

Professionals and all those who care about people with these difficult illnesses must understand that the illness has the power to change the perceptions of the environment. First-person accounts document the attraction that these altered perceptions may have for the patient. Because of the intensity and personal significance that may accompany the experiences of the illness, there may be a reluctance to give them up, and a real sense of loss when they are gone (MacKinnon, 1977). MacKinnon (1977) mourns the loss of his psychotic experiences:

I really missed my illness when I was free of it. I guess what I missed most was the sense of mystery. My visual hallucinations filled me with wonder and awe, as well as scaring me . . . . My illness was a great ego builder. Just think, God thought I was so special he was punishing me like this. It was quite a letdown to find that my "religious experience" was all a fraud and that people weren't really writing songs and magazine articles about me. (p. 427)

Houghton (1982) states that she has not relinquished the experiences of her psychosis, but carries them with her as a positive strength: "My first psychotic episode appeared as a private mental exorcism, ending with the honor of sainthood and the gifts of hope and faith. Fortunately, this sense of power became a source of tremendous strength during my recovery and sustains me even today" (p. 549). Another person's perception of the connection of the positive and negative sides of her experience is illustrated here:

> I have quite often experienced a euphoric "high" that is much like being in contact with some greater reality or meaning to life— accompanied by a kind of added brightness or extra dimension to everyday things around me. The other side of the coin, though, is a very intense anxiety from nowhere . . . . The two feelings are op- posite, yet somehow connected. Feelings are "the stuff life is made of," and I do not regret a lot of what I have experienced, but the terri- ble feelings are bad enough to make me opt for the medications . . . . (Anonymous, 1981a, p. 196)

Cognitive Confusion

Altered perceptions offer one distortion of the world and altered cognition, another. Andreasen (1984) has attempted to under- stand altered cognitive patterns by dividing them into four categories: (1) perceptual abnormalities, such as hallucinations; (2) thought content abnormalities, such as delusions; (3) inattentiveness and illogicality; and (4) formal thought abnormalities, such as poverty of speech content. She further distinguishes between perception and production of thought, concluding that the subject of thought disorder or cognitive confusion is one of the least understood terms in psychiatric illness. First-person accounts give a shadowy idea of what it is like to try to function with these illness-induced cognitive abnormalities (Andreason, 1984).

People in Freedman's study (1974) frequently described themselves with words such as confused, hazy, foggy, bewildered, and disoriented. Several patients reported thought blocking, which they described as their minds going blank or as a sudden loss of thoughts. Loosening of associations or being disconnected in speech shows the difficulty some patients have in tracking a particular idea. Sometimes the person starts a sentence or thought, but thinking veers off in another direction. The individual is unable to maintain cognitive con- trol (Anscombe, 1987).

My thoughts wander around in circles without getting anywhere. I try to read even a paragraph in a book, but it takes me ages, because each bit I read starts me thinking in ten different directions at once. (McGhie & Chapman, 1961)

_____

I couldn't read (newspapers) because everything that I read had a large number of associations with it. I mean, I'd just read a headline, and the headline of this item of news would have very much wider associations in my mind. It seemed to start off everything that I read, and everything that sort of caught my attention seemed to start off, bang-bang-bang, like that, with an enormous number of associations, moving off into things so that it became so difficult for me to deal with, that I couldn't read. (Laing, 1967)

Speech, as well as thinking, requires great concentration and conscious effort under these conditions of cognitive confusion. Leete (1987b) described this phenomenon when a flood of thoughts make her mute while she attempts to cope with them. Another person noted the following:

I "free associate" rather easily, and sometimes forget what I was saying because other ideas are in my mind. If I concentrate, however, this can be an advantage because I have a ready supply of new ideas . . . . Concentrating, though, is sometimes easier said than done. (Anonymous, 1981a, p. 197)

Responses may be predicated on illogical thinking as demonstrated here by Sechehaye (1951):

Mama brought me a gift—a little plush monkey of which I was at once afraid. When he had his arms up, I was anxious lest he hurt me . . . . Oddly, at that very moment, I felt the impulse to strike myself. I realized full well that my own arms were delivering the blows, still I was sure the monkey was attacking me. (p. 71)

Delusions and hallucinations are probably the best-known symptoms of mental illness. Torrey (1983) defines delusions as "false ideas believed by the patient and not by other people in his/her culture and which cannot be corrected by reason" (p. 24). These ideas have such salience for the patient that they endow them with a heightened sense of significance. The following first-person accounts illustrate this significance:

David was described as having a halo around his head, and the Second Coming was announced as forthcoming . . . . His mission would be to aid the poor and needy, especially in underdeveloped countries . . . . David believed that he was the only person who could prevent the impending war that would end the world. (Zelt, 1981, p. 528)

I believed that everyone was looking at me and I began sneaking down back stairways to avoid piercing looks. I could hear the low growl of a tiger following me. Eventually I believed my room to be electronically monitored and that my thoughts were being recorded . . . . I was sure the FBI was taking pictures of my every move. (Lovejoy, 1982, p. 606)

Leete (1987b) also described the experience of seeing the world as a series of messages to her—messages borne by car license plates or birds flying overhead. "Everything I see or hear is a direct message to me. The environment holds secret messages for me."

The messages may become complicated and may build on each other, creating symbolic thinking, as is illustrated in Bockes (1985):

On my way to school one day, three large birds soared over me, stalling briefly in the air above my head. In my class, I noticed a woman in front of me had a large black bag marked with white letters which read, among other things, "Urgent" and "Confidential." I heard a woman in the hallway say, "You won't go to jail." And my professor said during his lecture, "The choices you make are not inevitable," which angered and frightened me because I misunderstood him to mean, "The choices you make are inevitable." These events loomed in my head and I interpreted them as warnings of impending disaster. (p. 489)

Changes in Emotion

Emotions may rise or fall to abnormal levels in the course of the major mental illnesses (Hatfield, in press). Persons with schizophrenia and affective disorders may suffer from exaggerated feelings of fear and guilt, or from an absence of emotion. The loss of empathy with other people is one of the most troublesome aspects of mental illness. Such loss is particularly noticeable in the flattened emotions of some persons with schizophrenia. It is perhaps this emotional blunting that is most frustrating to mental health professionals who count on the building of reciprocal empathy with those people with whom they work. One mentally ill person describes the problem of intimacy:

Intimacy is an interesting problem in my life. In a way, I am capable of the deepest spiritual intimacy with people, yet I am less capable than most people of handling the demands of relationships. I cannot share negative feelings other people have, because I am too sensitive to them; yet I can give a great deal of love and concern when I am protected against feelings like anger and cynicism. (Anonymous, 1981a, p. 197)

Deep, severe, unrelieved depression may be the principal manifestation of the illness, or it may accompany the illness, as it sometimes appears to in schizophrenia. Depression may be a familiar emotion to the mental health professional, but the mentally ill person may experience it to a degree unknown to the professional, as the following account describes :

Being chronically depressed is like being trapped inside a bare, white room, a seamless monotony from which there is no escape. In fact, it is this which is the essence of depression: the despair of absolute nothingness, of being trapped in a complete void. Nothingness, that is depression—no color, no light, no spirit, no substance, no reality, no fantasy, just the paralyzing sense of despair that is nothing. *Absolutely nothing* can be done to change it." (Fish, 1985, p. 2)

Guilt is another emotion that may threaten to overwhelm the sufferer, as seen in this account of uncontrollable guilt:

I am haunted by a sense of guilt; my conscience gives me no rest, even when there do not seem to be any particularly grievous sins upon it. Whatever I am doing I feel I ought to be doing something else. I worry perpetually about my past sins and failure; not for a moment can I forget the mess I seem to have made of my life. However I may pray for forgiveness, no forgiveness comes. Eventually the terrors of Hell approach. (Custance, 1952, p. 61)

Torrey (1983) notes that patients often are subject to pervasive and nameless fears—fears that exist without any object. Fear can be one of the most disabling components of severe mental disorders. It may be immoblizing as the afflicted person seeks "a center of safety" (Landis, 1964) or it may lead to great agitation, as illustrated by Sechehaye (1951):

Suddenly Fear, agonizing, boundless Fear, overcame me, not the usual uneasiness of unreality, but real fear, such as one knows at the approach of danger, of calamity . . . . Outwardly, however, no one suspected the inquietude or the fear. People though I was hysterical or manic. (pp. 13, 14)

Severe mental illnesses bring with them the pain of changes in the sense of the self and in the sense of the body. It is no longer the known and reliable instrument but sometimes makes strange demands and is not always under its owner's control. The medications that control the illness and allow normal functioning exact a cost in their side effects, often changing how the body acts and feels to its owner. This is how a patient felt after discontinuing medication (Houghton, 1982): "My face was no longer swollen, extra pounds began to melt away; my hair grew thicker and more manageable; my movements were no longer mechanical and even my energy level increased" (p. 549). Bockes (1985) wondered if the medication caused her lethargy and inability to be involved in anything emotionally:

> Physically, I didn't feel too uncomfortable other than being stiff and "slowed down" most of the time, but what bothered me was my inability to get interested in anything, to be curious about anything, or to feel any emotion about anything. I often wondered if fluphenazine was causing my profound lack of interest and energy or if I was just being "lazy." (p. 488)

Leete (1987b) describes her conviction that she must take her medication to be "outgoing" and have a normal life. She then must deal with the *akathesia,* the irresistible physical restlessness that is a side effect of the medication.

The social self, the sense of the self that has hopes and goals, also changes as the mental illness makes itself inexorably known. The sufferer must cope with the loss of that self, and mourn that loss as one would the loss of a loved one. Leete (1987b) speaks of the growing self-image of the sick or ill individual, and how she mourns for that, and for what she might have become and accomplished. Stakes (1987) illustrates this dilemma:

> I now live a better life than I did at 20, but I would do better if I had no illness. Don't get me wrong. I live a good life, but I often wonder what kind of life I would lead without a disease of the mind. I have not given up hope of a successful life, but my lifestyle will always be attended by some dependency, primarily on medication. (p. 43)

Mental health professionals who can empathize with the grief that accompanies the recognition of the losses can be helpful to the sufferer in dealing with the mourning in all its guises. Mental health professionals who believe that the mental illness does not augur the end of all hope of a meaningful life and who are fully conversant with rehabilitation techniques and programs can help to settle the grief and turn the energy to setting new goals and reconstructing the sense of a meaningful life. This is described in Brundage's (1983) summation of a first-person account: "My illness has not meant the end of the world as I first thought, but it has opened a whole new world of personal resources for living and growing" (p. 585).

Discrimination

First-person accounts confirm that mental illness is accompanied by bewildering changes in the sense of self, as a direct result of the illness. Debilitating changes in the sense of self also are imposed as a result of the stigma that is associated with mental illness. Link, Cullen, Struening, Shrout, and Dohrenwend (1987) confirm that the stigmatizing process exists and that it has harmful effects. They found in a New York City study of stigma attached to mental illness that current patients, former patients, and nonpatients all agree that mental patients will be rejected by most people. They cite other studies that concluded that the term "mental illness" is one of the most highly rejected conditions, clustering with drug addict, prostitute, ex-convict and alcoholic rather than with cancer, diabetes, and heart disease. In the Link study, the stronger the mentally ill persons' belief that the mentally ill are rejected, the more likely their social networks were restricted to family and the more likely they were to employ coping strategies that included secrecy and withdrawal. Link et al. also found that those who were most strongly convinced that the label "mentally ill" was a stigma were the most likely to feel demoralized, to earn less income, and to be unemployed. Study subjects who exhibited significant pathology but were not labeled did not fall in the same pattern. Link and his co-authors suggest the possibility that the stigma experienced by those labeled mentally ill actually plays a role in the acquiring of deficit symptoms and may play a role in chronicity by leaving them in a vulnerable state. Leete (1987b) reflects that she learned the same feelings toward mental illness as everyone else. She says, "We grew up in the same society . . . it gives up our poor self image." Brundage (1983) describes her prejudice toward her disease:

> The stigma of mental illness was the hardest thing to overcome for me. I am embarrassed to admit how prejudiced I was. My attitude was, "It's o.k. for others, but it could never happen to me." It took me two years of intensive therapy, getting to know myself better, being fascinated, loving it and hating it, to accept what I am." (p. 584)

Leete (1987a) bluntly states that stigma is a negative factor in attempts to shape a normal life:

> An ever present obstacle keeping someone who has been psychiatrically labeled from reaching his or her potential is stigma.

There is nothing more devastating, discrediting and disabling to a person recovering from mental illness than stigma. In addition to the handicaps posed by our illness, we must constantly deal with the barriers erected by society. (p. 88)

In addition to the burden of estrangement that arises from the illness, there is the reality that the person labeled mentally ill is looked at differently from others, not just by general society, but by mental health professionals. Mental health professionals may avoid contact and interaction with those who have been severely ill. In addition to the stigma, mental health professionals may appear to have given up on certain patients. Leete (1987c) expressed this feeling:

Upon my return to the hospital I was met with silent anger. I sensed the staff were disappointed to see me again and that they secretly wished they would no longer have to deal with me. Naively I had expected that our relationship would be better if I returned voluntarily. I assumed that staff would see the evident change in my attitude and resume my treatment with the same optimism and energy I felt. (p. 488)

The scrutiny of every behavior for signs of illness presents a constant burden to anyone who has ever been labeled mentally ill. A psychiatrist, Daniel Fisher, who works with the mentally ill and who was himself mentally ill, speaks of the feeling when he is dressing for a professional appearance that he must look very "normal" (National Institute of Mental Health, 1986). Getting a job can be difficult and presents stresses unique to those who are stigmatized. When former patients are asked about whether they have ever received treatment, they are in a catch-22, as the following account illustrates:

If I were to be honest, as I naively was in the beginning, most assuredly I would never (and did not) hear from that interviewer again. If I discreetly manipulated my work history and possibly obtained the position, I might risk a future discovery and be liable for automatic dismissal . . . . There is much discrimination against people who seek or have obtained psychiatric treatment . . . . No matter how productive and functioning they are, the stigma is still there. (Anonymous, 1981b, p. 737)

Faced with a similar dilemma, Lovejoy (1982) notes the toll that was extracted from her abilities to function:

Applying for jobs far below my skills and intelligence, and fearful of discovery, I would become nervous and sleepless. If I complained to my doctor he would suggest perhaps I was not ready for work . . .

increase my medication, and I would suffer from blurred vision, sleepiness, further compounding my work problems. (p. 607)

Mental illness and menial occupations often fall together in our society, and the ill person feels a double discrimination, as Woodman's (1987) account points out: "The great majority of the staff there seemed to think that as I had a menial job, I must be a menial person. My feelings of loneliness increased there and started being accompanied by feelings of depersonalization" (p. 329).

To be like everyone else is a goal that the mentally ill seek, Godschalx (1986) concluded from interviews with people with **Community Living** long-term mental illness. Nothing about severe mental illness is easy, including a return to the community. Because the illnesses typically hit in early adulthood, education may be incomplete and there may be no established history of work. An established adult social network often is absent, whether one was never established or has disappeared, the person is faced with a void. Where to live, what to do, how to support oneself, where to find love and help, and who one can be are all questions with which one must deal. The social identity problem can be uncomfortable, as illustrated in the following accounts:

> If you meet somebody and they say what do you do all day and say I go to therapy and they look at you like you're nuts, and sometimes its hard to tell people that you go to therapy instead of work. They look at you funny. (Godschalx, 1986, p. 75)

> At a bus stop once, I struck up a conversation with a woman. The inevitable question arose: "What do you do?" I hestitated, but finally said that I was "retired" and that I had been in a psychiatric hospital. The woman's reaction was immediate and unforgettable. She gasped, then looked quickly for an approaching bus; seeing none, she flagged down a passing cab. (Lovejoy, 1982, p. 606)

Godschalx's (1986) interviewees want out of life what others want— home and family: "I want to get a nice car and a house and a wife." "I figure that if I had a little girl it would pull me through. I would have somebody to love and care for. I'm sure she would love me" (p. 68).

There are the fortunate persons who have been able to go back to an established niche, although adjustments may be made even there. An example is a physician whose residual illness prevented him from returning to the stresses of medical practice, but who found a congenial setting as a technician in a hospital dialysis unit (National

Institute of Mental Health, 1986). For those without an established niche, the creative and empathic mental health professional can play a critical role in working with the mentally ill person to discover and develop the alternatives that will bring about the sense of living like everyone else.

Practical Advice from the First-Person Accounts

The first-person accounts considered so far describe what the experience of being ill is like. They also can teach practical lessons of how to live with a life-disrupting illness. The accounts portray coping as well as suffering. The chronically mentally ill person experiences various internal and external phenomena, responds, and adapts. Those responses or adaptations may not be based on the same perceptions or logic as those of other people or as those of the mentally ill person at a different time. The accounts directly and indirectly suggest responses of professionals and of the mentally ill persons themselves that can be helpful. While hospitalized, the patients need continuity, acceptance, stability, silence, empathy, and routine. Once back in the community, they also need jobs, places to live, and the ability to cope with the illness' reoccuring symptoms.

Continuity of care is necessary to provide a range of services that can be used differentially based on the patient's condition. Leete (1987c) states: "Hospitals have their place in the treatment and stabilization of acute psychiatric problems. However, it is my opinion that long-term gains in functioning are made most readily and most successfully through treatment in the community" (p. 489).

It is in the hospital setting that mental health workers are most likely to meet and work with patients in their most acute stages. It is important that the mental health professional not stigmatize the person for actions taken when the person is coping with the illness in acute periods. Brundage (1983) notes: "Behavior while ill will need to be dealt with on the path to wellness" (p. 485). On the other hand, it is important for staff to acknowledge change in patients who have experienced difficult episodes, as reflected in the following account (Woodman, 1987):

> After about 3 weeks, I started feeling better, thanks to medication . . . . I started relating to less unwell patients. Still the staff left me alone. Didn't they know what was behind my illness? If they did they didn't let me know. I really just wanted to sit down and talk to somebody but could never find the right words. (p. 330)

First-person accounts suggest that during the difficult periods when the patient is experiencing altered perceptions and cognitive confusion, it is important for the environment to be stable:

> Because confusion and disorganization are primary characteristics, the patient can be helped by an atmosphere that is kind but firm, with expectations that are known. Explanations of treatment or of anything done to them or for them are essential . . . . Explain staff schedules. Explain, explain, explain! . . . Establish and maintain a daily routine and explain any variation of this routine. Setting limits provides security and at the same time encourages patients to reestablish their own limits. (Brundage, 1983, pp. 484, 485)

However, even routine activities may be difficult for the patient who is experiencing altered perceptions. Objects may not be integrated wholes and speech and sound may be fragmented. The worker needs to provide a consistent environment that is not contingent on the patient's ability to provide empathetic or verbal responses to the worker. The patient may need more time to respond than usual or may not be capable of verbalizing, as reflected in Brundage's (1983) account:

> Spend time with patients even when they are unable to respond verbally or in a seemingly incoherent manner. Silence is a communication tool that can be healing . . . . The proper environment can exert a vital force . . . . The enriched milieu can contain toxic overstimulation . . . . Sometimes the patient needs to withdraw and should be allowed to do so. (p. 485)

Mental health professionals, trained and accustomed to practice their craft in a highly verbal mode, can learn to recognize the cognitive stress of the illness, and modify their interactions. Brundage (1983) notes: "Everyone needs help sometimes; I happen to need help occasionally to think" (p. 585). Leete (1987b) describes the ways she controls her illness, providing clues for treatment to the professional. She limits distractions in the environment and gives herself time to make decisions. Professionals may need to give patients more time to respond at some points in their illness than at others. Explanations may need to be brief and concise, without extraneous information; the environment may need to be clear of distractions. Although chronically mentally ill persons may be trained to become more empathetic (Boston University, 1982), the mental health professional can facilitate interactions without demanding emotional reciprocity on the part of the client. The professional can recognize when the illness seems to bind the person's ability to react to others' feelings.

It is important for people both in the hospital and outside to understand what is happening to them. This can help to reduce the stigma attached to the illness. It can help to provide a sense of self-esteem and self-respect that are not only essential components of any therapeutic relationship, but help the patient to deal with the illness and its effects. Lovejoy's (1982) and Brundage's (1983) observations illustrate this point:

> The use of power which makes it possible for a handful of staff members to manage a ward also creates powerless victims, devoid of courage and self-respect. Power games create winners and losers; I was a loser . . . . Other patients especially understood my sense of shame, anger, and fear . . . . Although it helped to share experiences with others who genuinely understood, there were answers we could not give each other: how to overcome it all; how to make it on the outside. (Lovejoy, 1982, p. 607)

> Patients need to reaffirm that their feelings are valid and not so different from those of others under the same circumstances. (Brundage, 1983, p. 485)

This understanding may be necessary to help the patient deal effectively with the feelings generated by the illness, both as part of the symptomatology and as a result of the stigma attached to it.

But in addition to empathetic understanding is the need for knowledge, as underscored in this statement from Leete (1987c):

> Education about mental illness is crucial for everyone, but particularly for patients . . . . Patients and family members are entitled to education about mental illness, including its course, its treatment; more important, perhaps, they also need to know that the disease can be managed and there is reason to hope that the patient will live a satisfying and productive life. (p. 489)

Education about mental illness needs to be direct and to take into account the difficulties in learning and in attention that the patient may be experiencing. Opportunities for the chronically mentally ill person to formulate and to ask questions should be built into the educational process.

Hospital settings may provide routines for mentally ill persons more naturally than community settings; bureaucracies run on routine. The mentally ill person in the community faces many more choices and more chances that the outside environment will require adaptation than do those who are hospitalized. If the person is experiencing a chaotic or disrupted sense of perception or cognition, an imbalance of environmental demand and personal resources may be created. There are, however, routines that can help to provide the environmental structure that may be necessary to help the mentally ill person manage under pressure in community settings. The following account from Houghton (1982) illustrates methods to cope with the external stressors of community living:

> To maintain my sense of well-being, I have to change my lifestyle and my priorities. My illness has taught me (the hard way) the importance of meaningful work, good patterns of rest and sleep, exercise, diet, and self-discipline . . . a reasonable routine, a slower pace, and a calm atmosphere. I began . . . setting up a structure for everyday living. I put the schedule for "the ideal day" and "ideal week" in a small black notebook which I kept in my purse or briefcase. The notebook also stored . . . a running list of tasks to be accomplished. It reminded me what was important. (p. 549)

Leete (1987b) also uses her analysis of her past experiences with her illness to take control of the persisting illness. Her list of strategies for coping with the illness included items that kept her daily environment controlled, predictable, and low key. These strategies included writing a list of things to do; setting a predictable schedule, learning when to be alone and when to be with people, minimizing distractions, taking time to reach decisions and scheduling time between stressors (for example, social occasions). Leisure time presented particular problems for Leete. Because leisure time is unstructured, it can bring her close to panic. She therefore plans specific activities for leisure.

Work can provide structure in community settings. The mental health worker can be cognizant of some of the difficulties that may be involved in obtaining employment. However, the structure of a job can provide support to the mentally ill person who is living in the community, as illustrated in the following account by Leete (1987c):

> My job gives me something to look forward to every day, a skill to learn and improve, and an earned income. It is my motivation for getting up each morning, not always an easy task for psychiatric patients. My hours at work are passed therapeutically, as well as productively, for through steady employment I have learned to value myself and trust in my ability to overcome my disease. (p. 489)

The 1986 amendments to the Federal Rehabilitation Act mandate the provision of supported employment services for chronically mentally ill people in every state and may hold promise for many who have been lost to the everyday ordinary world of work. Besides income, work can provide a schedule, a place to go, a sense of accomplishment, and a sense of self-esteem.

Mentally ill people can be helped to develop techniques to manage mental states such as symbolic thinking and hallucinations. Leete

---

(1987b) reminds herself not to personalize observations of the environment. Bockes (1985) used the following tactics when faced with her own symbolic thinking:

> I spent several hours . . . thinking and writing in my journal, and I arrived at two basic conclusions: (1) that by trying to ward off whatever calamity seemed to be approaching, I would inevitably bring on a calamity of my own creation by acting prematurely; and (2) that perhaps I'd noticed them in order to justify my growing fear . . . . No disasters occurred. (p. 488)

Bockes further suggests that recognizing those things over which she has control or some control is useful. She notes that

> there are a few things over which I have little or no control—i.e., hallucinations. The trick is to realize when or if the hallucinations are truly disrupting my thoughts, feelings, and behavior, and to take appropriate action by using medication before things get out of control. (p. 489)

Thus, medication management is a coping strategy that can be used with patients monitoring their perceptions and behaviors. It is important for patients to recognize that the value of the medications outweighs the nuisance of side effects (Florke and Kjenaas, 1987).

From first-person accounts emerges the world of mental illness, a world that is individual, exciting, and frightening. Mental health professionals need knowledge, understanding, and empathy for the experiences of mentally ill people so that they can develop treatment that responds to the diversity and range of client perceptions and behaviors. Basic empathy provides the basis for relationships that acknowledge illness and expand the ability to cope.

References

Andreasen, N. (1984, July 20). Concepts of thought disorder said confusing. *Psychiatric News,* pp. 17, 24.

Anonymous. (1981a). First person account: Problems of living with schizophrenia. *Schizophrenia Bulletin, 7,* 196–197.

Anonymous. (1981b). The quiet discrimination. *Schizophrenia Bulletin, 7,* 736–738.

Anscombe, R. (1987). The disorder of consciousness. *Schizophrenia Bulletin, 13,* 241–260.

Bockes, Z. (1985). First person account: "Freedom" means knowing you have a choice. *Schizophrenia Bulletin, 11,* 487–489.

Boston University. (1982). The skills of psychiatric rehabilitation videotape series: Teaching a skill. Boston: Center for Psychiatric Rehabilitation.

Brundage, B. E. (1983). First person account: What I wanted to know but was afraid to ask. *Schizophrenia Bulletin, 9,* 585–586.

Carpenter, W. T. (1986). Thoughts on the treatment of schizophrenia. *Schizophrenia Bulletin, 12,* 527–539.

Custance, S. (1952). *Wisdom, madness, and folly.* New York: Pellegrini & Cudahy.

Fish, G. (1985, September). *What it's like to be chronically depressed.* [Indiana Community Support Network News]. Indianapolis: Indiana Department of Mental Health.

Florke, B., & Kjenaas, M. A. (1987). *The videotape guide* (Understanding and coping with mental illness videotape series). Cherokee, IA: Community Psychiatric Services Unit, Mental Health Institute.

Freedman, M. A. (1974). Subjective experiences of perceptual and cognitive disturbances in schizophrenia. *Archive of General Psychiatry, 30,* 333–340.

Gladstein, G. A. (1983). Understanding empathy: Integrating counseling, developmental, and social psychology perspectives. *Journal of Counseling Psychology, 30,* 467–482.

Godschalx, S. M. (1986). Experiences and coping strategies of people with schizophrenia. Unpublished doctoral dissertation, University of Utah.

Hatfield, A. (in press). *Helping families with mentally ill relatives: An educational approach.* New York: Guilford.

Hogarty, G. E., Anderson, C. M., Reiss, D. J., Kornblith, S. J., Greenwald, D. P., Javna, C. D., & Madonia, M. J. (1986). Family psychoeducation, social skills training, and maintenance chemotherapy in the aftercare treatment of schizophrenia. *Archives of General Psychiatry, 43,* 633–642.

Houghton, J. F. (1982). First person account: Maintaining mental health in a turbulent world. *Schizophrenia Bulletin, 8,* 548–549.

Kaplan, B. (Ed.). (1964). *The inner world of mental illness.* New York: Harper & Row.

Laing, R. D. (1967). *The politics of experience.* New York: Ballantine Books.

Landis, C. (1964). *Varieties of psychopathological experience.* New York: Holt, Rinehart & Winston.

Leete, E. (1987a). A patient's perspective on schizophrenia. In A. B. Hatfield (Ed.), *Families of the mentally ill: Meeting the challenges* (pp. 81–90). San Francisco: Jossey-Bass.

Leete, E. (1987b). *Strategies of coping* (Understanding and coping with mental illness videotape series). Cherokee, IA: Community Psychiatric Services Unit, Mental Health Institute.

Leete, E. (1987c). The treatment of schizophrenia: A patient's perspective. *Hospital and Community Psychiatry, 38,* 486–491.

Link, B. G., Cullen, F., Struening, E., Shrout, P. E., & Dohrenwend, B. P. (1987). A labeling theory approach to mental disorders: An empirical assessment. Unpublished manuscript, University and New York Psychiatric Institute, New York.

Lovejoy, M. (1982). Expectations and the recovery process. *Schizophrenia Bulletin, 8,* 605–609.

MacKinnon, B. L. (1977). Psychotic depression and the need for personal significance. *American Journal of Psychiatry, 134,* 427–429.

McGhie, A., & Chapman, J. (1961). Disorders of attention and perception in early schizophrenia. *British Journal of Medical Psychology, 34,* 103–116.

McGrath, M. E. (1984). First person account: Where did I go? *Schizophrenia Bulletin, 10,* 638–640.

Minor, D. (1981). Third side of the coin. *Schizophrenia Bulletin, 7,* 316–317.

National Institute of Mental Health. (1986). *Employing the skills of the mentally restored: A roundtable discussion* [Videotape]. Bethesda, MD: National Institute of Mental Health.

Schreber, D. P. (1955). *Memoirs of my nervous illness.* (I. Macalpine & R. A. Hunter, Eds. and Trans.). London: Dawson.

Sechehaye, M. (1951). *Autobiography of a schizophrenic girl.* New York: New American Library.

Stakes, M. (1987). Becoming seaworthy [Special Issue]. *Schizophrenia Bulletin, 13,* 43–44.

Strauss, J. S. (1986). Discussion: What does rehabilitation accomplish? *Schizophrenia Bulletin, 12,* 720–723.

Torrey, E. F. (1983). The inner world of madness. In *Surviving schizophrenia: A family manual* (chap. 2). New York: Harper & Row, p. 5–44.

Woodman, T. (1987). First person account: A pessimist's progress. *Schizophrenia Bulletin, 13,* 329–331.

Zelt, D. (1981). First person accounts: The messiah guest. *Schizophrenia Bulletin, 7,* 527–531.

HEALTH ISSUES AND AFRICAN-AMERICAN WOMEN:
Surviving but Endangered
Audreye E. Johnson

I'm sick and tired of being sick and tired.

These words of Fannie Lou Hamer, spoken in the midst of the fight to gain simple liberties in Mississippi and throughout America in the 1960s, remain a part of the legacy of African-American women. The burden of womanhood in America is a shared experience of all women, but for African-American women it has its roots in the peculiar institution that placed an added load to the gender role—racism. Depending on her health, age, and economic status, the African-American woman may move beyond double jeopardy to triple, quadruple, or quintuple jeopardy, but at all times she remains in double jeopardy. Therefore, one can be African-American, female, poor, old, and in ill health.

The "African-American Civil Rights Renaissance Movement" of the 1960s influenced many groups to look more closely at their status within American society. These people either revitalized their organizations or began new ones, freely borrowing without appreciation many of the tactics of the movement. Women were very much a part of efforts to make changes during this period, as they had in the past. For African-American women, their double jeopardy raised questions regarding where their energies should be placed. As has been a part of the history of African-Americans, regardless of gender, these women did not have the luxury of a single-item agenda or of finding self through work. A.E. Johnson (1987a) and Marshall (1987) noted that the African-American woman has been dually disenfranchised, African-American women were considered chattel because of race and sex, and did not have rights because of their gender, and all women were not seen as citizens.

The past has influenced the present for African-American women. Their health status has been impacted by the barriers of race, gender, age, and poverty. Moreover, these factors have in part determined their caregiving and nurturing role within their community. Some selected issues that have critical relevance for the physical and mental well-being of African-American women are presented in this article.

Roots of Discovery

African-American women, whether free or enslaved, began making formal individual and organizational contributions to African-American progress and self-help through their church activities, their support of the abolitionist movement, and the establishment of independent female groups as early as the eighteenth century. These activities were documented by Aptheker (1971), Jackson, Rhone, and Sanders (1973), Quarles (1969), Ross (1987), and Wesley (1969). Obviously, the family has been an ongoing institution where African-American women have nurtured their people and participated in their community's development. The activities of African-American women's contribution to their community and people have been in concert with their African-American brothers, but also have been independent of them. The multidimensional role of African-American women not only began early but was further solidified during the development of women's clubs in the nineteenth century. The main goal of these clubs was the uplifting and improvement of the African-American community. These women moved through all spheres of the population, from the cradle to the grave, providing many social work and social welfare services.

Despite such stellar behavior, little attention was given to the African-American woman as an entity in her own right until the 1970s. Hoytt (1986)) noted that the "birth of Black women's studies was in 1970 with Toni Cade's anthology on Black women, but it came of age in 1982 when the work *All the Women Are White, All the Blacks Are Men, But Some of Us Are Brave: Black Women's Studies* (Cade, 1970) was published" (p. 28). Those scholars, such as Ladner (1971), Lerner (1973), and Staples (1973), who early began to address the African-American woman, recognized the race, sex, or economic issues of oppression faced by African-American women but not the other jeopardies of age and health. More recent works have continued in this vein or have sought to make clear the difference between oppression faced by African-American women and by Caucasian women, or the racism operative within Caucasian women as they join Caucasian males in the oppression of African-American women and men (Chafe, 1978; Daniels, 1970; Davis, 1981; Dill, 1979; Giddings, 1985; Harley & Terborg-Penn, 1978; Hooks, 1981, 1985; Rodgers-Rose, 1980; Sterling 1979, 1984).

Concern regarding women's health issues began to emerge in the 1970s. Ruzek (1986a) noted the struggles at the onset to place women's health courses within academia and the slowness of attention to cultural and ethnic issues related to this type content. She stated:

> The first type of course that entered the academy was what can be termed a "body course," modeled after self-help courses offered in the community. Historically, these are the hardest to track and trace, because they were often taught at the margins of the academy by temporary, part-time faculty in women's studies programs or under the sponsorship of a faculty member who wouldn't, couldn't, or was afraid to teach such a course. Some in fact were student-taught and carried group study or independent study credit under the sponsorship of a sympathetic faculty member. Because they often were carried out under special study titles, and only entered the college catalogue later, historians will have to rely on archival material and oral history to date their "beginnings" accurately. (p. 10)

Elsewhere, Ruzek (1986b) discussed the myths, biases, and difficulty in teaching about minority women's health. The need to be aware of the health issues related to women of color to be sensitive to their needs and to adequately "reflect more accurately the very nature of health and illness" (p. 35). In further delineating the rationale for teaching and integrating minority content into health courses, she stated, "When we consider the experience of minority women we may develop a very different view of what constitutes health and illness, health seeking behavior, and the history of health care than if we exclude minority women from our consciousness and our scholarly work" (p. 36).

One group that has sought to address health content regarding women of color is the Women, Health and Healing Project of the University of California at San Francisco. This project has produced summer institutes and developed and published bibliographical and course content materials. The relevance of this type of content for social work education was noted by A. E. Johnson (1986) in the design of a graduate course. The resource material of the project (Clarke, Olesen, & Ruzek, 1986; Ruzek, Anderson, Clarke, Olesen, & Hall, 1986; Ruzek, Olesen, & Clarke, 1986) covered different disciplines related to health issues and recognized the diversity related to women in both a general and a specific sense.

Recognition of the health issues facing African-American women led to a conference, Black Women's Health Issues, held in June 1983 in Atlanta on the campus of Spelman College. The success of this first national conference was an enabling force in the continuation of the National Black Women's Health Project in Atlanta. Moreover, affiliates have been established in other locations with an ongoing focus on the health and wellness of African-American women. Local conferences have been held that have focused on the concept of self-help in the wellness of African-American women. This recent organization encourages taking responsibility for one's own health through familiarity with one's body and its functions, and has garnered support from diverse groups of African-American women. In addition to holding conferences, this group publishes a newsletter, *Vital Signs*. On May 31, 1987, a film developed by the organization premiered, entitled "On Becoming A Woman: Mothers & Daughters Talking Together."

The search for a framework within which to examine the African-American woman becomes essential to understanding her and the barriers she faces in American society. The importance of the African perspective in viewing African-Americans has been articulated by several scholars. Some scholars who have noted and presented evidence of the persistent "presence of African thinking, behavior, and life style . . . among American Blacks, Billingsley, Blassingame, Gordon, Jackson et al., Jones, Ladner, Thompson, and White are just a sampling of these scholars" (A. E. Johnson, 1987b, p. 8). Recognizing the differences that exist between African-Americans and others as well as those present within the black community has value for understanding and increasing one's knowledge regarding a people. An African-American perspective gives due recognition to the converging influences of African, European, and American cultures on Negroid people in the United States, resulting in an Afro-Euro-American life content. In this point of view African-Americans are not filtered through a Caucasian American perspective, but are valued for their own uniqueness. Terborg-Penn (1987) argued for an "African Feminist" framework because "through the 'White filter' the lives of Black women are viewed from the outside-in, rather than from the inside-out" (p. 4). The health issues facing African-American women can be understood and appreciated best when viewed from an African Feminist perspective.

African-American Women

The health of African-American women is affected by their biological, psychological, and social well-being. This is in line with the World Health Organization's definition of health. Behavior or life-style, however, also is a determinant of one's health status. In summary, health is influenced by individual, family, and societal conditions, or stated another way by socioeconomic status and position. The question arises: What are the bio-psychosocial variables that interact and influence the health of African-American women? African-American women have been victims of societal restrictions related to citizenship opportunities and availability of resources that have interacted in a negative manner to deny or curb their access to modern health care. The barriers related to health care for people have been noted by Watkins and Johnson (1985).

The technological advances in medicine, knowledge, and opportunities for leisure living have combined to positively affect the health and life span of all Americans. The change in the life expectancy of African-Americans in this century has more than doubled. "By 1982, . . . life expectancy [for blacks] averaged 69 years (65 years for men and 74 years for women), about 6 years less than Whites" (D. L. Johnson, 1986, p. 12). African-American women share with other women gender longevity; in 1980 women accounted for 51.4 percent of the total population (Dion, 1984). African-American women made up 52.7 percent of the African-American population in 1980. This has particular reference for African-American women who are more likely to be widowed before retirement and find it necessary to work to support themselves and possibly significant others. For those 65 years and older, women make up 59.7 percent of the population. Although people are living longer, it also must be noted that African-Americans continue to be a young population group. The median age of African-American women in 1982 was 26.8 years, compared with 24.1 years for African-American males and 31.6 years for all Americans. These data indicate that many African-American women will never marry or have children, but may well become the caregivers within their group to family members and significant others.

It is not only that African-American women outlive their male counterparts, but the age when this begins to happen is quite significant, that is, 15 years. This early date has meaning for the life-style and general well-being of African-American females. Work becomes a necessity not only because of the differential wage paid to African-Americans and Caucasians—in the instance of married couples, both must work. African-American women may have to work for self-support and possibly for the support of aged or sick parents. The differential of African-American women with other women widens greatly when looking at the male and female mortality figures. The decline in the male populations of Caucasians does not begin until age 35 which is a 20-year difference; for other minorities of color and those of Spanish origin, women begin to outnumber males at age 25, a 10-year difference (Dion, 1984).

The marital status of African-American women and those of Spanish origin for 1982 were as follows: 29.6 percent were single, 47.3 percent were married, 13.5 percent were widowed, and 9.6 percent were divorced. The husbands of these women were likely to be African-American (U.S. Bureau of the Census, 1983). The median family income for blacks in 1984 was $15,430. Only 29 percent of African-American families had incomes of $25,000 or more. "Stated another way, for every $100 a White family received, a Black family received $56" (D. L. Johnson, 1986, p. 6). To earn a middle-class income, African-American women usually work. Hill (1987) noted:

> Yet, working couples continue to be the backbone of the Black middle-class. While married couples comprise three-fifths of all Black families, they account for four-fifths of middle-class families. And Black wives are more likely to work than White wives— regardless of class position. Three out of five Black wives work, compared to only one out of two White wives. In fact, the strongest economic gains relative to Whites occurred among Black couples with two wage earners. (p. 32)

The poverty level of African-Americans has continued to be higher, ranging from 32.5 percent in 1980 to 33.8 percent in 1984. The rising number of female-headed households accounts for much of this increase in poverty. African-American women are the lowest paid wage earners—median 1984 income was $8,650—and usually have children or others dependent on their scarce earnings. According to D. L. Johnson (1986), "Black female householders accounted for 73 percent of all poor black families in 1984" (p. 6).

The work ethic runs deep in the African-American community, but the results of racism, sexism, and unequal screens of opportunity have colluded to rebuff efforts for advancement, especially among African-American women. The growth of women in the work force has been consistent. Dion (1984) reported that "women now constitute 43 percent of the entire labor force of the Nation, and are responsible for nearly 60 percent of its growth since 1970" (p. 7). The majority of women continue to work in traditional occupations. For African-American women, this means that the largest group of employed women are in clerical (24.6 percent) and service (28.6 percent) positions, with a spread in other occupations from technical (3.1 percent) to machine operators (12.7 percent). African-Americans made up 19.2 percent of social workers in 1980, 61,547 of whom were black women (Matney & Johnson, 1984).

Living longer has not led to a better life-style for African-Americans. Older African-Americans in 1980 were almost 8 percent of the African-American population. Wheeler (1986) reported that "research on how Black people age, both physiologically and psychologically, has been a lonely and not particularly prosperous endeavor over the past decade" (p. 5). The elderly African-Americans have been the fastest growing segment of the African-American population with an increase of 34 percent during the 1970s. The majority of African Americans has been economically below the middle-class income level in their working years, and remain economically strapped in their later years. Nearly 40 percent of the African-American elderly live in poverty. Continuing to be on the lowest rung of the economic ladder in old age has been the plight of African-American women. It has been noted that among those with incomes below the poverty level are "three out of ten Black female family householders 65 and over" (Dion, 1984, p. 12).

Selected Health Issues

The recent *Report of the Secretary's Task Force on Black & Minority Health* (U.S. Department of Health and Human Services [HHS], 1985) called dramatic attention to the disparity of African American minority illness and death with the nonminority population. Particularly, there was concern regarding the excess deaths and higher incidence of major illness in African-American and minority health. The report not only pointed out the problems, but made recommendations that would decrease the existing disparity. Money expenditure was only one of the things that needed to be done. Also of importance was sensitivity in attitude of health care practice professionals, policymakers, program implementors, and administrators, and access, availability, and accountability of consumers and providers. The task force made eight recommendations related to the following six specific areas: (1) health information and education, (2) the delivery and financing of health services, (3) health professions' development, (4) cooperative efforts with the nonfederal sector, (5) data development, and (6) research agenda. The report also examined mortality in the African-American community:

EXCESS DEATHS expresses the difference between the number of deaths actually observed in minority group and the number of deaths that would have occurred in that group if it experienced the same death rates for each age and sex as the White population. (p. 63)

The six causes of death found by the task force to account for more than 80 percent of excess mortality among African-Americans were (1) heart disease and stroke, (2) homicide and accidents, (3) cancer, (4) infant mortality, (5) cirrhosis, and (6) diabetes. "For Black males and females combined, excess deaths accounted for 47 percent of the total annual deaths in those 45 years old or less, and for 42 percent of deaths in those aged 70 years or less" (p. 4). When looking at African-American female deaths, the excess rate can be seen to be significantly higher than those for Caucasian females—631.1 rate per 100,000 population for blacks compared with 411.1 for Caucasians (p.67). The average number of excess deaths for each disease category for African-American females yearly is shown in Table 1.

Cornely (1970) found that African-Americans tended to have a lower death rate after about age 75. This idea was picked up by the task force, which stated in the report:

In later life, minorities have lower death rates for many diseases than do nonminorities. This "survior effect," or mortality crossover, has been attributed to hardiness among survivors in a population that has a higher early-age death rate (p. 74).

African-Americans under age 45 are at relative risk for other diseases as well (Table 2). Deaths from TB and anemia, although not major causes of death, occur at a higher frequency among African-Americans and may be related to socioeconomic conditions commonly associated with these diseases (HHS, 1985).

Three diseases that are reported to be prevalent among African-American females are hypertension, diabetes, and anemia. African-American women were two times more likely to have these diseases than Caucasian women. "These morbidity figures clearly show the health disparities in Blacks surfacing early in life, and several health conditions responsible for the disparities are known risk factors for cardiovascular disease" (HHS, 1985, p. 75).

Until recently, the power brokers have given little attention to the African-American community in connection with the disease that has invaded the total world population—acquired immune deficiency syndrome (AIDS). This disease has disproportionately affected the African-American community in America. Unfortunately, the impression has been left that again the ugly heads of discrimination and

Table 1
Excess Deaths by Disease for African-American Females

Disease	Under Age 45		Under Age 70	
	Excess Deaths	% of Total	Excess Deaths	% of Total
Cardiovascular	1,416	17	9,712	41
Cancer	424	5	2,269	10
Cirrhosis	419	5	782	3
Infant mortality	2,861	35	2,861	12
Diabetes	107	1	1,203	5
Unintentional injuries	-86	0	134	1
Homicide	1,145	14	1,381	6
All other	1,848	22	5,203	22
Total deaths	8,220	100	23,545	100

SOURCE: HHS, 1985, p. 71.

racism have been busy sowing their seeds of exclusion. There have been negative accusations regarding AIDS based on the number of cases in Africa, and subsequently, the blaming of African-Americans for the disease. The barriers of homophobia and the insensitivity to people of color in the decision-making nonminority community has caused the African-American community to be ignored. This has been especially damaging to African-American women.

Fortunately, the African-American community has not been remiss in making some effort to disseminate information and educate the populace regarding this disease. Getting information to the African-American community about the disease has been left largely to black community leaders. The National Urban League, in its 1987 *State of Black America,* reported on AIDS. The Joint Center for Political Studies also dealt with AIDS in its publication *Focus,* and both *Ebony* and *Essence* magazines have run feature articles on AIDS in the African-American community during 1987 and 1988. The Office of Minority Health, Public Health Service, sponsored a small meeting of community leaders of people of color in June 1987. A national forum to discuss AIDS and people of color was sponsored by the Centers for

Table 2
African-Americans at Relative Risk of Death by Disease

Disease	% Males	% Females
Tuberculosis (TB)	17.4	15.6
Hypertension	10.2	13.4
Homicide	6.6	4.3
Anemia	6.0	5.2

SOURCE: HHS, 1985, p. 75.

Disease Control in August 1987. This slow movement has been regrettable in light of the fact that African-Americans comprise 25 percent of the AIDS cases but are only 12 percent of the population. Of all homosexually or bisexually transmitted AIDS cases, 14.64 percent are African-American. African-Americans also account for 51 percent of all intravenous (IV) drug-related AIDS cases, and for 22 percent of cases that involve people who are homosexual or bisexual and are also IV drug users. African-American women account for 51 percent of all female AIDS cases. More than half of the AIDS cases in the African-American community are among heterosexuals. *Newsweek* (Staff, 1987) reported the startling statistic that "the census of the dead stands at 22,548 now, by the government's conservative count. As many as a million and a half more Americans are thought to be infected with the AIDS virus . . . one responsible estimate is that the body count will have reached 179,000 by 1991" (p. 22).

African-American women are getting AIDS from their sexual partners and from the use of contaminated or shared needles in IV drug use. These women are having babies who are already infected with the disease, which will in turn further affect the infant mortality rate in the African-American community. Although there is no cure for AIDS (and only limited treatment now exists), the disease has no boundaries related to race, sex, socioeconomic status, or age. Additionally, AIDS as well as other diseases affect not only the bodily function but the psychological and social aspects of life.

Education is one of the chief means of combating AIDS, but because of the concentration of attention on Caucasian male homosexuals, myths have been perpetuated that now must be undone. The focused attention on the male homosexual has resulted in the majority of groups offering information regarding the disease being controlled by Caucasian gays and lesbians. This has presented barriers to caring and communication about the disease in the African-American community. Unfortunately, racism and sexism remain a part of the life experience and life-style of the Caucasian homosexual.

Homosexuality has been taboo behavior in the African-American community. Codes of conduct transmitted from Africa became part of the Afro-Euro-American life experience. Gutman (1976), Hare and Hare (1986), Nobles (1986), Thompson (1974), and White (1984) noted that African traditions and codes of behavior remained viable and were adapted as a part of the culture and life-styles of African people in America. This legacy has inhibited African-Americans from admitting the changing life-styles and values that came from the blending of their African and European heritages. The AIDS threat made it easy for African-Americans to deny the disease in their community based on their African history of shunning homosexuality. The mass media hype provided credence to this view by highlighting AIDS as a Caucasian male homosexual disease. African-Americans had ignored the growth of homosexuality and bisexuality in their community, and initially lacked information regarding AIDS and its connection with IV drug use. African-American women, in support of their families and community, have kept the myths of sexual behavior intact by refusing to acknowledge the existence of their man's relationships with other females or other males.

Given the history of mistreatment by the medical community, trust is not easily given by African-Americans to modern medicine. Past experimentation and brutal surgical episodes remain vivid in the African-American community to be passed along on the "grapevine." The reality of this type of treatment has been noted by Axelsen (1985), Cope and Hall (1985), Jones (1981), Morais (1976), and Watson (1984). Education regarding AIDS in the African-American community needs to be sensitive to the values and cultural perceptions of the people. The historical thought process of African-Americans related to homosexuality and experimentation by the medical profession will need recognition and careful handling.

The ongoing paucity of African-American health professionals is another barrier to be overcome. Especially for African-American women there have been greater obstacles to securing a medical education. The absence of role models has been the result of this type of discrimination and racism. the history of African-American women in health care education has been well documented by Hine (1985a,b).

Implications for Social Work

Some of the life issues that face African-American women, making them vulnerable to the jeopardies of race, gender, age, poverty, and health problems, have been presented here. The past cannot be ignored when attempting to provide social work service to African-American women. Many of the health problems that they face are a part of their history of exclusion within American society. The trust level is another important aspect that has to be addressed. The peculiar institution of the past has made trust difficult. Therefore, social workers and other service providers need to be sensitive to the cultural background of African-American women, keeping in mind the diversity that exists within this group. The African-American experience has been and is diverse, as are the screens of opportunity.

African-American women are confronted with a series of problems over their life span, as noted by the report on black and minority health (HHS, 1985). Health problems begin at an early age and continue through old age. Such problems affect functioning and socialization within the family, community, and society and may well affect self-concept. The low income paid to African-American women is another barrier to securing or seeking necessary health care. The attitude of the health professionals whom African-American women encounter may become another barrier to the health-seeking process. Answers must be sought to overcome previous inequities to access in health care and health information, keeping in mind that the distrust harbored is based on reality, not fantasy.

Many health problems confront the African-American woman, but currently the disease that is running unchecked throughout society is AIDS. This disease threatens the core of the African-American community—the family. Ignorance can be dangerous to the health of the African-American community, but especially to the African-American woman. The African-American woman is the incubator for populating the African-American community, and so, if her health or that of her fetus or newborn is at risk, the African-American community could be annihilated.

Education is necessary if the disease is to be in check until a cure can be found. The fears that have run wild in society will have to be overcome if preventive education regarding AIDS is to occur. Social work through the National Association of Black Social Workers and the National Association of Social Workers (NASW) have made a start in addressing AIDS in their conferences. Additionally, NASW has published a book related to working with AIDS patients (Leukefeld & Fimbres, 1987).

While continuing to function as caregivers in their community, African-American women need to focus on their own health. African-American women will need to become more involved in taking charge of their health by becoming familiar with their body functions to make accurate health decisions and to avoid neglect. Their sensitivity to discussion of personal issues, even with friends, will have to be overcome. African-American women will need to be supported to alter their learned secret behavior and resultant discomfort regarding the discussion of personal issues in general, and health issues in particular. This cultural pattern generates a wall of silence and allows health problems to go unchecked. Improved communication within and without the group will be important. Change is called for on all sides, but health professionals will have to take the lead with knowledge, understanding, and respect for difference. Moreover, demonstrating sensitivity to the African-American woman and her wall of silence will help to reduce this barrier.

The stress of being African-American and female in America has been constant. From the wider society, the African-American woman has been abused as a nonperson, sexual object, and a matriarchal figure of super-human strength; unfortunately, some within the African-American community buy into this unwarranted propaganda. All of these terms and behaviors are detrimental to a real view of the African-American woman and depreciate her. More research is needed on how the African-American woman has survived and remained functioning with resilience to be an asset to the African-American community. Her supportive, nurturing, and caregiving qualities should be put in proper perspective, a partnership deal with the African-American community.

With acumen, the African-American woman has managed to balance the biopsychosocial aspects of her life. While much more is needed, she has managed to continue the struggle for more than survival in a hostile environment, keeping ahead of the various risks from illness, disease, poverty, socioeconomic status, racism, and sexism in performing her tasks and roles with the African-American family, community, and society at large. The present risks to health threaten the African-American female and menace functioning at her best potential.

The African-American woman is intertwined with all of American society, not just the black community. Failure to recognize and address the collectivity of this existence in facing common enemies of pestilence, meager health care, and discrimination is to invite continued separation as well as mutual health problems. Social work can contribute to the improved health of African-American women and of society through a more sensitive and appreciative approach to understanding African-American women.

References

Aptheker, H. (Ed.). (1971). *A documentary history of the Negro people in the United States* (Vol. 1). New York: Citadel.

Axelsen, D. E. (1985). Women as victims of medical experimentation: J. Marion Sims' surgery on slave women, 1845-1850. *Sage, 2,* 10–13.

Cade, T. (Ed.). (1970). *The black woman: An anthology.* New York: Signet.

Chafe, W. H. (1978). *Women and equality.* New York: Oxford University Press.

Clarke, A., Olesen, V., & Ruzek, S. (Eds.). (1986). *Teaching materials on women, health, and healing.* San Francisco: Women, Health and the Healing Program, University of California.

Cope, N. R., & Hall, R. R. (1985). The health status of black women in the U.S.: Implications for health psychology and behavioral medicine. *Sage, 2,* 20–24.

Cornely, P. B. (1970). Community participation and control: A possible answer to racism in health. *The Milbank Memorial Fund Quarterly, 48,* 347–362.

Daniels, S. I. (1970). *Women builders* (rev. ed.). Washington, DC: Associated Publishers.

Davis, A. Y. (1981). *Women, race and class.* New York: Random House

Dill, B. T. (1979). The dialectics of black womanhood. *Signs, 4,* 543–555.

Dion, M. J. (1984). *We, the American women.* Washington, DC: U.S. Government Printing Office.

Giddings, P. (1985). *When and where I enter: The impact of black women on race and sex in America.* New York: Bantam.

Gutman, H. G. (1976). *The black family in slavery and freedom, 1750–1925.* New York: Vintage.

Hare, N., & Hare, J. (1986). *The endangered black family: Coping with the unisexualization and coming extinction of the black race.* San Francisco: Black Think Tank.

Harley, S., & Terborg-Penn, R. (1978). *The Afro-American woman: Struggles and images.* Port Washington, NY: Kennikat.

Hill, R. B. (1987). The black middle class defined. *Ebony, 1052,* 30–32.

Hine, D. C. (1985a). Opportunity and fulfillment: Race and class in health care eduation. *Sage, 2,* 14–19.

Hine, D. C. (1985b). Black women physicians in America: The pioneers, 1865–1925. In R. Abrams (Ed.), *Send us a lady physician: A history of the American woman in medicine, 1825–1925.* New York: Norton.

Hooks, B. (1981). *Ain't I a woman: Black women and feminism.* Boston: South End.

Hooks, B. (1985). *Feminist theory: From margin to center.* Boston: South End.

Hoytt, E. H. (1986). Integrating feminist issues into curricula at historically black colleges. In A. C. Clarke, V. Olesen, & S. Ruzek (Eds.), *Teaching materials on women, health and healing* (pp. 24–31). San Francisco: Women, Health and Healing Program, University of California.

Jackson, W. S., Rhone, J. V., & Sanders, C. L. (1973). *Social service delivery system in the black community during the ante-bellum period (1619–1869).* Atlanta, GA: Atlanta University School of Social Work.

Johnson, A. E. (1986). Syllabus on African-American women's health issues. In A. Clarke, V. Olesen, & S. Ruzek (Eds.), *Teaching materials on women, health and healing* (pp. 99–107). San Francisco: Women, Health and Healing Program, University of California.

Johnson, A. E. (1987a, March). *The black experience workshop—1987.* Final program statement for the Eighth Annual Black Experience Workshop, Chapel Hill, NC.

Johnson, A. E. (1987b, June). *The movers and the shakers: African-American women and social welfare development.* Paper presented at the Annual Meeting of the National Women's Studies Association '87, Atlanta.

Johnson, D. L. (1986). *We, the black Americans.* Washington, DC: U.S. Government Printing Office.

Jones, J. H. (1981). *Bad blood: The Tuskegee syphilis experiment—a tragedy of race and medicine.* New York: Free Press.

Ladner, J. (1971). *Tomorrow's tomorrow: The black woman.* Garden City, NY: Doubleday.

Lerner, G. (Ed.). (1973). *Black women in white America: A documentary history.* New York: Vintage.

Leukefeld, C. G., & Fimbres, M. (Eds.) (1987). *Responding to AIDS: Psychosocial initiatives.* Silver Spring, MD: National Association of Social Workers.

Marshall, T. (1987, May 30). Speech made May 6, 1987, at the Annual Seminar of the San Francisco Patent and Trademark Law Association, Maui, HI. *The Carolina Times,* pp. 1, 11.

Matney, W. C., & Johnson, D. L. (1984). *America's black population: A statistical view, 1970-1982* (Special publication P1O/POP-83-1, Bureau of the Census). Washington, DC: U.S. Government Printing Office.

Morais, H. M. (1976). *The history of the Afro-American in medicine.* Cornwells Heights, PA: Publishers Agency.

Nobles, W. W. (1986). *African psychology: Towards its reclamation, reascension & revitalization.* Oakland, CA: Black Family Institute.

Quarles, B. (1969). *The Negro in the making of America* (rev. ed.). London: Macmillan.

Rodgers-Rose, L. (Ed.). (1980). *The black woman.* Beverly Hills, CA: Sage.

Ross, E. L. (1978). *Black heritage in social welfare, 1860–1930.* Metuchen, NJ: Scarecrow.

Ruzek, S. (1986a). Women's health studies in the United States. In A. Clarke, V. Olesen, & S. Ruzek (Eds.), *Teaching materials on women, health and healing* (pp. 8–16). San Francisco: Women, Health and Healing Program, University of California.

Ruzek, S. (1986b). Integrating minority women's health into the curriculum. In A. Clarke, V. Olesen, & S. Ruzek (Eds.), *Teaching materials on women, health and healing* (pp. 35–43). San Francisco: Women, Health and Healing Program, University of California.

Ruzek, S., Anderson, P., Clarke, A., Olesen, V., & Hall, K. (Eds.). (1986). *Minority women, health, and healing in the U.S.: Selected bibliography and resources.* San Francisco: Women, Health and Healing Program, University of California.

Ruzek, S., Olesen, V., & Clarke, A. (Eds.). (1986). *Syllabi set on women, health and healing: Fourteen courses.* San Francisco: Women, Health and Healing Program, University of California.

Staff. (1987, August 10). The face of AIDS. *Newsweek,* 22–39.

Staples, R. (1973). *The black woman in America: Sex, marriage, and the family.* Chicago: Nelson-Hall.

Sterling, D. (1979). *Black foremothers: Three lives.* Old Westbury, NY: Feminist.

Sterling, D. (Ed.). (1984). *We are your sisters: Black women in the nineteenth century.* New York: Norton.

Terborg-Penn, R. (1987). Theories for researching and writing black women's history. *Truth: Newsletter of the Association, 9,* 4.

Thompson, D. C. (1974). *Sociology of the black experience.* Westport, CT: Greenwood.

U. S. Bureau of the Census. (1983). *Statistical abstract of the United States: 1984* (104th ed.). Washington, DC: U.S. Government Printing Office.

U.S. Department of Health & Human Services. (1985). *Report of the Secretary's task force on black & minority health* (Vol. 1). Washington, DC: U.S. Government Printing Office.

Watkins, E. L., & Johnson, A. E. (Eds.). (1985). *Removing cultural and ethnic barriers to health care* (reprint). Chapel Hill, NC: Schools of Public Health & Social Work, University of North Carolina at Chapel Hill.

Watson, W. H. (Ed.). (1984). *Black folk medicine: The therapeutic significance of faith and trust.* New Brunswick, NJ: Transaction.

Wesley, C. H. (1969). *Neglected history: Essays in Negro-American history by a college president.* Washington, DC: Monumental.

Wheeler, D. L. (1986, October 29). Neglected issue of aging among blacks needs more study, researchers warn. *The Chronicle of Higher Education,* p. 5.

White, J. R. (1984). *The psychology of blacks: An Afro-American perspective.* Englewood Cliffs, NJ: Prentice-Hall.

RURAL SOCIAL WORK: Addressing the Crisis of Rural America

O. William Farley, Kenneth A. Griffiths, Mark Fraser, and Lou Ann B. Jorgensen

The problems of rural America seem to be evident in all parts of the United States. Farmers are caught in the vicious inflation–disinflation cycle when they discover that the value of their land is not equal to the debt they owe. Interest rate gyrations and low product prices add to the economic plight of rural America.

In the western areas of the country, the erstwhile energy boom brought tremendous population growth in the late 1970s and early 1980s. The boom soon turned into bust as the price of oil dropped drastically; rural boom communities found themselves bust communities, with high unemployment and social deterioration.

There are many problems in rural America that need to be solved. The social work profession can provide important leadership in the area of social services if it takes a proactive stance with local communities and their leaders. Social workers with an environmental focus prepare others in the profession philosophically and methodologically to address and ameliorate many of the problems found in rural America.

Castle (1985), in his last presidential address for the organization Resources for the Future, stated:

> During the past three decades some rural communities have been emptied of most of their people and now confront a crumbling social infrastructure. Others have had to cope with enormous growth when a manufacturing plant has located nearby, or when they come within commuting distance of an urban center. This rapid change in the numbers and composition of the rural population makes it difficult to plan for the needed investment in social services and may destroy, at least temporarily, the sense of community that is critical both to group decision making and the quality of life. (p. 4)

Rural communities are struggling to exist. More and more evidence is coming out of rural America to substantiate the deepening crises. Majors (1985) illustrates the crisis:

> Not since the 1930s have we seen such an economic recession in the farm sector. The "farm crisis" is real as across the nation we see farmers and their families uprooted from land by bankruptcy while small rural communities are dying . . . . Farm families are suffering emotionally—husband, wife and children. A "family farm" means just that—involvement of each member of the family—in the production, decisions and emotional involvement.
>
> Historically, farm families have been very stable, but we are beginning to see the results of the stress affecting many families. We are seeing mental breakdowns, divorce, farm accidents, suicides, abuse, both verbal and physical, as families are losing their farms. Children and teenagers are showing the stress. (p. 5)

Several studies and papers (Albrecht, 1982; Hefferman & Hefferman, 1986; Jacobsen & Albertson, 1987; Joslin, Emerson, & Rossman, 1986) have documented the increase of stress in farm families, increased depression and withdrawal from the community, increased stress-related illnesses, and increased disturbances in family functioning, including marital problems and parent–child conflicts.

The entire structure of many rural communities seems to be seriously threatened. Fitchen (1987) stated: "The challenge for human service agencies and community institutions in rural America is indeed tremendous. The financial and personnel resources for meeting that challenge are already stretched too thin . . ." (p. 56).

Study Background

Recognizing the growing problems of rural America, the Social Research Institute (SRI) at the Graduate School of Social Work,

University of Utah, conducted a series of studies in rural communities to identify problems and ways of mitigating those problems.

The first study was an attempt by SRI staff to find out what social service management strategies had helped rural social workers and social work administrators cope with the problems of both boom and bust conditions. To find out what really worked, 38 rural social service practitioners who had been living and working in rural areas were given a detailed and lengthy management strategies analysis form containing 532 specific strategies statements. The top 40 management strategies were identified from this study, and form a guide to effective social work practice and administration in rural areas.

The second study grew out of the management strategy studies. One of the areas important in managing problems in rural areas is to conduct meaningful needs assessments. The needs assessment process provides an important tool for the rural social worker. The completed needs assessment provided additional evidence of the problems confronting rural communities. The needs assessment included a sample of 416 individuals who had lived through both the boom and bust phenomena in three rural counties of Utah.

Both of these studies illustrate the kind of planning and focused activity that will be required of rural social workers. The results of the two studies are presented in this article in a summarized form. It is hoped that studies of this nature will assist rural social workers in their attempts to mitigate the increasing problems of rural America.

Management Strategy for Mitigating Rural Social Problems

The social work profession cannot really impact many of the forces causing the problems in rural America. However, the profession can do a better job of planning and managing sparse resources that mitigate rural problems and needs.

Based on the premise that the profession can find a better way to manage social service in rural areas, SRI set out to discover what planning and management techniques worked best for social service providers in rural areas of Utah.

In preparation for the actual study, the research staff reviewed current literature to identify critical social service management strategies. Major studies suggested important basic management areas that must be addressed by any rural social service agency. From the literature review, the research team identified the following eight management categories that then guided the study:

1. Data collection and utilization
2. Planning

3. Funding
4. Staff support
5. Service coordination
6. Client access to services
7. Special agency services
8. Community consultation and education

After the major categories were identified, further literature searches assisted the research team in the development of 15 to 60 specific strategy statements under each of the eight categories. The specific statements were critical in the development of this project because the research team believed it was important to have an instrument that was clear and understandable. The instrument provided practitioners with the opportunity of rating to what extent they used the strategy and how effective it was in managing rapid population shifts. The instrument also provided the research team with some specific and quantifiable data.

Because the management strategy analysis forms (MSAFs) contained 532 variables, the data from the practitioner sample were collected on a group basis. The research team met with 38 social service personnel in three rural areas, gave group instructions regarding the MSAF, and remained in the room to offer consistent interpretation and help as needed.

The MSAF was designed with a seven-point Likert scale that provided a numerical score on each of the specific management strategy statements. Through a unique scoring process (utilization mean + effectiveness mean/2 = grand mean), the research team identified the top five strategies in each category, which are described in this chapter.

As the social service professionals finished each section of the MSAF, research staff members tallied their responses to each management strategy and identified the strategies used most frequently and judged most effective (grand mean) in each of the eight major categories. These strategies were then listed on newsprint, and the personnel in the groups discussed how they used each of the highly used strategies in dealing with the rapid population changes in their respective areas. These group discussions were productive in clarifying specifics—what social service personnel did to mitigate social service problems, and how they did it.

Findings

This section presents the findings of the study. Each of the top five strategy statements are presented as recommendations to social service directors along with a summary of the professional group discussion that took place during the process.

The findings of this category suggest that social service directors collect data on individuals, groups, classes, and seminars regarding types of services provided and **Category 1— Data Collection and Utilization** number of clients served. Additionally, social service directors should report all service data to the public through the association of governments, compare growth in service demands to population shifts, obtain and utilize data from industry in making service projections, and monitor growth in service demands as any new industry begins its start-up process.

The discussion supported the notion that one of the most important tasks in the process was use of the management infor- *Professional Group Discussion* mation system designed by the Utah State Department of Social Services. It was noted that there were many improvements that could be made in the system. Examples were given regarding the need for data summaries to be more accessible to local units and more relevant to local situations. Also identified was a need for local units such as industries, schools, law enforcement, and social service units to share data. A final suggestion was to create a uniform data collection system throughout all state social service divisions.

Another strategy supported by the group discussion was the need to continually document service delivery episodes. These data could then be used to report to units of government, such as county commissioners, associations of governments, and advisory boards. The groups also pointed out that baseline data from social service agencies were critical in facilitating comparisons in service demands as population shifts occurred or as new industries developed. These data were not available in any of the areas at the outset of energy development.

The groups indicated that during the early periods of the boom cycle many industries were reluctant to share their basic projection data with social service units. In some instances, industries provided inaccurate or incomplete data. It was suggested that social service personnel find ways to gather accurate projections from industry.

Also discussed was the tendency of many data collecting entities to fail to project important "at-risk" populations. One of the populations that was not projected properly was that consisting of transients who have little or no work skills. This group needs special attention in all stages of growth (for example, rapid, stable, and decline).

The findings of this category suggest that social service directors communicate agency needs to state and county governments, consider community values in planning, work with county commissioners to coordinate and plan for human services, and use prevention planning, especially for high-risk populations.

**Category 2—
Planning**

The groups recognized the need for social service units to continually communicate agency needs to county and state governments.

*Professional
Group
Discussion*

It was felt that social service units often become so busy in providing direct service that they neglect the communication and coordination planning that is essential for their long-term effectiveness. The professional groups were consistent in recommending the establishment of regular (at least monthly) meetings to report planning activities, service data, and program needs to units of government, including state legislators. The necessity of such planned meetings relates to all eight management categories, and is one of the strongest recommendations identified by the professional group for mitigating the impact of population change.

The group felt the items referring to the need to consider community values in planning and prevention planning for high-risk populations are also critical to the mitigation process. Again, these two areas can easily be neglected under the pressure of providing direct service.

One of the important findings of this discussion was the fact that social service personnel believe they need a designated planner either from within their own system or from the state system. One discussion group was adamant that the planner needs to be from the local area to fully consider community values in planning. Another group was equally adamant that the planner should be an outsider, so that he or she could be totally objective and not become involved in "turf battles" between agencies when funding is considered. Whether insider or outsider, all recognized the use of a designated, full-time planner as essential to the planning process.

It was suggested that the designated planner have the ability to assimilate and use data in accessing funding sources. One group believed that the designated planner from the state level was able to offer needed assistance because of his or her understanding of funding sources.

It was agreed that one of the most important tasks the designated planner must assume is the creation and use of local councils. The groups stressed the importance of involving community members at all levels on the advisory councils. The advisory council may be linked to or empowered by the association of governments in the area. The importance of using advisory councils was consistently emphasized in the discussions. These councils were identified as being vital power brokers for the social service agencies as they work to meet the unusual needs of rapidly changing populations.

According to group opinion, a third role of the designated planner is to be sensitive to county commissions. The sense of the discussion reinforced the notion that credibility must be established between the county commissioners and social service programs if services are to be effective in the community and that human service directors should give high priority to keeping government officials well informed of service activities, needs, and problems.

Category 3— Funding

The findings of this category suggest that social service directors write special grant proposals for private and government agency support, use statistical information to support funding needs, have regular planned meetings with state and local government officials to present needs and request funding, monitor ongoing funding needs in the agency, and use needs assessment and program evaluation data to support funding requests.

Professional Group Discussion

As the funding management strategies were analyzed, it became apparent that rural agency social service providers need a staff person who is specially trained in grant writing, or that such technical assistance should be readily accessible through state agencies. The group was aware that funding needs are the lifeline of the small social service agency and require constant attention, and that many rural communities are penalized because they lack the expertise necessary to compete successfully for available grant funds.

Group discussion reemphasized the need to have staff people within the agency who have both the skill and the interest to write grant proposals. Actually, the three sites in the study reported that they have been successful in providing funds for both extra staff and for services.

While many of the strategies from data collection, planning, or funding overlap, the groups stressed again the importance of basing all funding requests on a solid data base, and determined that funding needs must be monitored by social service agencies. The group believed the monitoring process must be shared regularly and realistically with important local and state officials as well as with advisory councils.

The findings of this category suggest that social service directors use in-house staff support through regular case staffings, **Category 4— Staff Support**

communicate appreciation to staff and acknowledge work well done, use in-house staff support through group training sessions, emphasize the hiring of experienced staff, and provide flexible or individual staff scheduling.

The group recognized that staff pressure increases as service needs increase in small communities, and that under these circumstances staff support management *Professional Group Discussion*

strategies such as in-house training, open communication, recognition of quality performance, and flexible scheduling would assist in alleviating and managing the stress associated with increased demands for service. The rural social service providers suggested the need for employing experienced people because of the variety of roles the worker must perform.

One subject that engendered a lot of discussion was the need to streamline hiring practices. Social service staff faced with increased service needs could remedy this situation by being able to hire people more quickly and in a more flexible manner. One group suggested that state social services might develop an impact team of trained workers who would be willing to move into an area on a temporary basis and assist local staffs until regular hiring processes could be implemented.

The groups also expressed the need for providing increased monetary incentives for individuals to work in rural areas. They made the point repeatedly that rural social service work requires a person who can assume a very difficult "generalist" role. This role is made more difficult when the boom phenomenon occurs.

All three groups agreed that regular weekly and as-needed daily staffing of cases helped staff to support one another, and that interactions around such items as assessment and treatment interventions were very helpful. Staff members also identified interagency staffing, where roles were defined and mutual treatment plans were formulated, as being of great value.

A flexible and individualized work schedule was recognized as an important stress-reducing mechanism for social services personnel. Some staffs worked four 10-hour days, then took three days off; others rotated shifts and responsibilities.

A final strategy discussed by the groups to reduce staff pressure was the establishment of an on-call duty roster to cover evening/weekend emergencies. Apparently the rotated on-call provisions protected social service workers from having to deal with constant emergency pressures. When the duty roster was extended to include personnel from all the social service agencies in the community, it was even more effective.

Category 5—Service Coordination

The findings of this category suggest that social service directors use the colocation of agencies to facilitate service coordination between agencies, a voluntary human service council for information sharing, an interagency directors' council to coordinate services between agencies, child protection teams to coordinate services between agencies, and an association of government-sponsored human service committees to provide recommendations regarding coordination of resource allocation.

Professional Group Discussion

Respondents believed that colocation of agencies, coordinating councils, and child protection teams helped with service coordination, and that although smaller communities have excellent potential for service coordination, it must be continually and purposefully orchestrated. They felt that as a community is impacted with rapid population growth or decline, the need for service coordination becomes more acute and that service coordination must include community agencies other than those ordinarily under the social service umbrella, such as law enforcement and churches.

The professional group discussions reaffirmed that service coordination is facilitated by colocation of agencies. Such things as client and staff convenience, easier communication, and positive information interaction were suggested as being very important. Examples of negative elements of colocation were client labeling and difficulties arising from unified funding.

The agency director's role in service coordination was identifed by the group as being very important. They felt that agency directors in the area need to schedule regular meetings at least monthly to coordinate their services. Three specific tasks suggested for the directors' meetings were (1) elimination of duplication of services between agencies, (2) coordination of interagency on-call duty rosters, and (3) planning for needed community volunteer service.

Also discussed was the state-mandated child protection team. The group members stated that the child protection team, which included key individuals from the schools, law enforcement, youth correction, and the Office of Community Operations (OCO), was effective and important in service coordination.

Transients were identified as a particularly difficult group to include in coordinated services. Two of the three areas reported that they had finally worked out a very formal and structured transient referral service that included key people from law enforcement, churches, and OCO. Group consensus was that a key element in the system was the designation of one agency person in the community to coordinate all transient services. Every agency in the community would refer transients to one person, thereby eliminating duplication of services.

Category 6— Client Access to Services

The findings of this category suggest that social service directors use on-call duty rotation for after-hour client contact, colocate with other human service agencies, provide marriage and family counseling, make home visits, and create an information and referral system within the community.

Professional Group Discussion

It was suggested that an after-duty call roster was very important in providing client access to services. The respondents again ranked colocation high on the list of strategies for providing good client access. Two unique strategies suggested were the need to make home visits and to create an information and referral system within the community. Finally, the notion that marriage and family counseling needed to be offered in rural agencies to facilitate client access reinforces the fact that many rural individuals and families are in need of these services.

The professional group discussions reinforced the singular importance of an after-hours, on-call duty roster for social service agencies in boom and bust areas. Workers recognized the need for client access, especially in the late hours. They also pointed out the necessity for outreach through home visits to clients, especially to elderly, handicapped, and isolated individuals.

The findings of this category suggest that social service directors provide individual therapy, implement a crisis line, initiate preschool programs for the developmentally disabled, provide outpatient therapy for victims and perpetrators of domestic violence, and provide family therapy for spouse abuse.

Category 7— Special Agency Services

The respondents indicated that in any community undergoing population change, the social service agency must continue to provide individual and family therapy. The need for a crisis line was also highly rated.

Professional Group Discussion

Discussion data indicated that many of the special agency service needs were centered on individual and family therapy for problems in the area of domestic violence. The three groups reported that they had experienced increases in child and spouse abuse as their communities had gone through the boom and bust stages.

Another special service mentioned was the development of sexual trauma teams to deal with problems of incest and rape. Concern was expressed that staffs were not properly trained in this area, and that rural areas do not have enough resources to deal with these types of problems.

The findings of this category suggest that social service directors use advisory boards of lay citizens, politicians, and human service providers, develop educational programs in parenting skills and in communication skills, encourage multipurpose use of social service and recreation facilities, and develop educational programs in stress management.

Category 8— Community Consultation and Education

In analyzing the community education and consultation strategies, it was obvious that respondents believed educational programs focused on parenting skills, communication skills, stress management, depression, battered/battering spouses, elderly, adolescents, and substance abuse were all important in population-impacted areas.

Professional Group Discussion

The use of a strong advisory board and the offering of both social service and recreation facilities to multiple use seem to be important to mitigation. Group discussion centered on the need for using advisory boards consisting of lay members as well as representatives of human service agencies, law enforcement, churches, the planning office, associations of governments, schools, news media, the Utah Congress of Parents and Teachers, service clubs, and others who are aware of community needs. The need for such boards to be responsible for keeping the community informed and supportive of social service funding needs was recognized. Respondents indicated the importance of agency visibility in the community.

The group noted the importance of budgeting for education and recreation for newcomer integration and for prevention. One agency reported budgeting $5,000 annually for county recreation, which guaranteed the director a position on the county board and provides exposure to county leaders who can lend support to social service agencies.

The 40 top ranked strategies identified by our study of 38 rural professional administrators and workers form the nucleus of an effective mitigation approach that can assist rural social workers. A simple but hopefully effective social service field guide that can be used by rural social workers in guiding their practice was developed from these strategies.

Needs Assessment: Protocol and Findings

Recently, there has been a growing awareness that individuals living and working in a community know the human service needs of the community and that collectively they can give planners a realistic basis on which to develop programs. The needs-assessment process is a well-accepted procedure that provides quantifiable data on the perceptions of community residents. The perceptions of the residents can then be prioritized and used as the focal point of community discussions. Such discussions tend to build consensus between community residents, social service personnel, and community leaders. Thus, the needs-assessment process facilitates effective social service program planning and implementation (Austin, 1987).

A review of the needs-assessment literature was undertaken to assist in the design of a needs-assessment protocol and instrumentation package. It was decided that four different populations should be included in the study. The study populations were:
1. Community residents
2. Social service providers
3. Community leaders
4. Native American community leaders

Questionnaires were developed for each of the study populations. The questionnaires were completed and field tested by January 1, 1986. Data collection occurred between January 1, 1986, and June 1, 1986. Each study population was sampled in a slightly different fashion and the questionnaires were tailored to each group; however, there was enough commonality built into the process to allow for intergroup comparisons. The community residents, social service providers, and community leader populations included Caucasian, Indian American, Hispanic American, Asian American, and black American community members in numbers that are representative of the ethnicity of the community.

Review of the writings of authorities on social needs assessment indicates that the most comprehensive and reliable needs-assessment data are acquired when residents, community leaders, and social service workers contribute their perceptions of need to the database. Researchers worked conscientiously to achieve this end. Data were provided by a random sample of 230 residents and a purposive sample of 64 social service workers, 19 community leaders, and 17 leaders of the native American tribe. Recognizing that the native American people could benefit from identifying their needs within a tribal frame of reference, a sample of 97 members of the tribe also provided data pertinent to the study. Because the tribal member schedule was developed using a different format, the data are only directly comparable in certain instances. It is appropriate that these data are specifically identified and included in this paper. The major data, however, come from the 330 residents, leaders, and providers interviewed in the basic study. Two important areas were selected for this presentation—suggestions for urgent service expansion and identification of community problems.

Suggestions for Urgent Service Expansion

Respondents were asked to weight on a seven-point scale the urgency of a list of human service needs—1, not needed, to 7, extremely urgent. Only those who responded that the needs for such services were very urgent (5) to extremely urgent (7) were included in the data presented in Table 1. All of the 5, 6, and 7 responses were totaled to determine an urgency score that provides a cumulative weighting of all respondents' perceptions of urgency of service needs.

It is almost inconceivable that 185 of the 330 respondents (57 percent) would identify the need for child/spouse abuse counseling as the most urgently needed service in the community. The second highest urgency score of 1,051, for a residential center for adolescent alcohol

Table 1
Rank Order of Services Urgently Needed as Identified by Four Groups of Uintah Basin Respondents

Services to be Expanded	Residents	Providers	Leaders Non-Indian	Leaders Ute Tribe	Total Number	Mean Urgency Ratings[a]	Urgency Score[b]	Rank
Counseling services for child and spouse abuse	126	39	9	11	185	6.13	1,134	1
Residential center for adolescent alcohol and drug	114	34	3	12	163	6.45	1,051	2
Support group for single parents	106	33	10	9	158	6.0	948	3
Residential center for adolescents with emotional problems	107	31	5	11	154	6.03	929	4
Counseling in hospitals for emotional problems	91	41	6	8	146	5.96	870	5
Residential center for adults with emotional problems	84	24	5	10	123	6.03	742	6
Mental health service close to home	49	22	4	12	87	5.9	513	7

[a]The mean urgency rating is the mean score for all urgent to extremely urgent responses (5, 6, and 7) on the seven-point urgency scale.
[b]The urgency score is calculated by adding all urgent to extremely urgent scores (5, 6, and 7) on the seven-point urgency scale.

and drug treatment is impressive in and of itself, but when one considers that the fourth most urgently needed service (urgency score 929) is for a residential treatment center for adolescents with emotional problems, the need for an intensive treatment unit for youth is staggering. There are obviously some very serious problems among the communities' youth that are not being appropriately treated through existing out-patient services.

Recognizing the high cost of residential treatment would suggest the need for establishing close service ties and program agreements with residential adolescent treatment centers in the urban areas of Utah. It may be more appropriate to use available funds for achievable service expansion in child/spouse abuse counseling (top urgency score 1,134), support groups for single parents (948), and counseling for emotional problems in hospitals (870).

Community Problems

Respondents from the four sample groups were provided several different ways to identify the social/emotional problems and needs of their communities and residents. One of the most effective ways was to provide respondents with a list of common human problems and ask them to indicate how frequently they observed or had knowledge of each problem and ranked its seriousness on a seven-point scale. The serious (5) to extremely serious (7) scores were then cumulated to determine a mean seriousness rating that could be multiplied by the number of respondents giving a rating of 5, 6, or 7, and arrive at a total weighted seriousness score. These data combined for the four sample groups are presented in Table 2.

Unemployment and financial problems rank first and second in seriousness in the minds of the total respondent group identifying these problems as serious to very serious. Alcohol/drug problems rank third in seriousness, with 181 of 330 respondents rating this problem as serious to very serious. If drug abuse, which ranks eighth in the seriousness score, is combined with alcohol problems, this combined total again becomes the most serious problem. Engaging in such combinations changes the order only slightly. With all sample groups and in the combined format, the same broad problems clearly emerge among the top five: (1) job and economic problems; (2) alcohol and drug problems of adults and youth; (3) lack of constructive leisure time programs and facilities; (4) marriage, family, youth, child conflict/violence; and (5) personal stress, anxiety, depression, and loneliness problems. The seriousness rating in Table 2 provides a more definitive breakdown of each category of need; but to address them programmatically, there seems to be some rationality to grouping

Table 2

Rank Order of Serious to Extremely Serious Ratings of Problems by Four Groups of Uintah Basin Respondents

Problem	Residents	Providers	Leaders Non-Indian	Leaders Ute Tribe	Total	Mean Seriousness Ratings[a]	Seriousness Score[b]
Unemployment	153	40	16	17	226	6.33	1,431
Financial problems	145	26	17	16	204	5.86	1,195
Problems with alcohol	116	35	13	17	181	6.10	1,104
Problems of raising children	100	39	8	11	158	5.98	945
Stress or anxiety	99	33	11	10	153	5.90	903
Depression	93	31	7	7	138	5.83	805
Family conflict	84	29	11	13	137	5.85	801
Drug abuse	73	33	8	13	127	5.93	753
Teenage problems	83	23	10	9	125	5.80	725
School problems	68	28	8	14	118	5.80	684
Juvenile delinquency	72	20	10	13	115	5.78	665
Marital conflict	69	24	9	10	112	5.68	636
Crime	66	29	4	7	106	5.90	625
Loneliness or isolation	64	25	6	10	105	5.86	615
Poverty	58	14	5	9	86	5.65	486
Chronic mental illness	46	9	4	8	67	5.68	381
Sexual abuse	38	13	4	11	66	5.53	365
Physical violence	38	17	2	7	64	5.48	351
Problems of senior citizens	35	11	4	7	57	5.50	314
Eating disorders	34	3	3	11	51	5.65	288
Suicide	25	14	2	8	49	5.80	284
Chronic physical illness	23	13	3	6	45	5.72	257
Physically handicapped	20	17	3	3	43	5.18	244
Child abuse	19	11	1	8	39	5.75	224
Mental retardation	8	2	1	1	12	6.73	81

[a]The mean seriousness rating is the mean score for all serious to extremely serious responses (5, 6, and 7) on the seven-point seriousness scale.

[b]The seriousness score is calculated by adding all serious to extremely serious scores (5, 6, and 7) on the seven-point seriousness scale.

them. For example, a program that provides a total family, child, and youth prevention/treatment programmatic thrust could address many of the specific needs identified in Table 2.

As we try to become too discrete, we lose the broader vision of commonality of problems and perhaps lose efficiency in the use of limited resources. It may be that the greatest hope for addressing the extremely serious human needs of community residents in times of increasing need and decreasing resources will require a move away from overly individualized service to more broadly focused educational/prevention/self-help/individual and group-support networking service programs.

The summarized needs assessment presented indicates that rural residents in Utah perceive themselves and their communities as having serious financial, emotional, and family problems. If this urgent sense of need for social service planning and assistance is not addressed, the stage might very well be set for Castle's prediction—that a "sense of community" may be destroyed. Communities must respond to the needs of their citizens to maintain the quality of life in rural communities.

Currently, the needs-assessment analysis is being presented to the three counties involved in the study by rural social workers. Social workers are sharing the findings with both community leaders and residents. The consensus and priority-setting processes are well underway. The communities seem to accept social work leadership and ideas when social workers present a thoughtful needs assessment to them. The needs-assessment process is an important tool for the rural social worker.

Proactive Social Work Leadership

The problems and struggles of rural America are going to continue well into the next decade. Rural social workers have the skills to mitigate many of the problems. The two studies summarized in this article hopefully can be used as both process and content guidelines in actual rural practice. The management strategies are important guides to rural social work directors. These guidelines can assist social service agencies to effectively plan for and use scarce resources.

The needs assessment that grew out of the management strategies study is currently being used as a focal point for community planning. The top five problems of (1) job and economic problems, (2) alcohol and drug problems of adults and youth, (3) lack of constructive leisure time programs and facilities, (4) marriage and family problems, and (5) personal stress and anxiety and depression are being addressed by the community. The urgency and sense of pervasiveness of problems expressed by the rural residents is motivating the communities to use their resources in more effective ways to mitigate their problems.

In both of these two studies, rural social workers played critical roles. They demonstrated strong proactive leadership bringing professionals, politicians, and community leaders together in a positive and productive problem-solving mode. While the rural social worker may not be able to effect an upturn in the economy or create new jobs, he or she can mitigate individual, family, and community stress by skillful planning and managing to assure that communities are continually working to solve their needs.

References

Albrecht, S. L. (1982). Empirical evidence for community disruptions. *Pacific Sociological Review, 23,* 297–306.

Austin, D. M. (1987). Social planning in the public sector. In A. Minahan, R. M. Becerra, S. Briar, C. J. Coulton, L. H. Ginsberg, J. G. Hopps, J. F. Longres, R. J. Patti, W. J. Reid, T. Tripodi, & S. K. Khinduka (Eds.), *Encyclopedia of social work* (18th ed.; pp. 620–625). Silver Spring, MD: National Association of Social Workers, Inc.

Castle, E. N. (1985, September 30). The forgotten hinterlands: Rural America. In *Annual report 1986* (pp. 2–10). Washington, DC: Resources for the Future.

Fitchen, J. M. (1987). When communities collapse: Implications for rural America. *Human Services in the Rural Environment, 11,* 56.

Hefferman, W. D., & Hefferman, J. B. (1986). Impact of the farm crisis on rural families and communities. *The Rural Sociologist, 6,* 160–170.

Jacobsen, G. M., & Albertson, B. S. (1987). Social and economic change in rural Iowa: The development of rural ghettos. *Human Services in the Rural Environment, 11,* 58–65.

Joslin, F. J., Emerson, L. A., & Rossman, M. R. (1986). Mental health response to farm crisis victims. In *Proceedings of the Rural Mental Health Conference* (pp. 171–184). Omaha: University of Nebraska School of Social Work.

Majors, B. (1985, Fall). A new perspective on the farm crisis. *Commission Quarterly,* p. 5.

TREATING MARITAL COUPLES IN CONFLICT AND TRANSITION

Donald K. Granvold

Behavioral marital therapy (BMT) has become established as a major model of marital treatment through the pioneer efforts of such clinician–reseachers as Jacobson and Margolin (1979), Liberman (1975), Rappaport and Harrell (1975), Stuart (1975, 1980), and Weiss (1978). The BMT methods of these and other empirically based clinicians have continued to receive the careful scrutiny of controlled research. As a result of these ongoing efforts, there has been an evolution in BMT to include a consideration of cognitive and affective variables. This trend to include the assessment and treatment of cognitive variables also has been paralleled in the treatment of a host of other disorders including depression (Beck, Rush, Shaw, & Emery, 1979), anxiety, phobias, and stress disorders (Michelson & Ascher, 1987), bulimia (Hawkins, Fremouw, & Clement, 1984), anger (Novaco, 1975), children (Meichenbaum, 1977), and sexual dysfunction (Emery, Hollon, & Bedrosian, 1981).

The integration of cognitive processes in BMT and conceptual tenets of cognitive–behavioral marital therapy (C–BMT) are discussed, and procedures for engaging couples in treatment are presented in this article. Faulty information processing and irrational beliefs and expectations are explored as they relate to marital interaction.

The approach to the treatment of marital problems described here incorporates the application of social learning and behavior exchange principles with cognitive assessment and intervention methodology. Although in an embryonic stage, C–BMT can be expected to provide a valuable new dimension to the treatment of marital distress.

Conceptual Tenets of Marriage and Marital Treatment

The theoretical foundation of BMT was derived from empirically validated principles of learning. Although BMT and other behaviorally oriented therapies showed promising results, the limited power of learning principles to explain intricate contextual and subjective variables became apparent (Guidano & Liotti, 1983). To reduce the discrepancy between theory, techniques, and ongoing clinical observations, the conceptual base was expanded to include cognitive factors. The emerging conceptual base of C–BMT examined in this section reflects the influence of learning theory blended with cognitive domains relevant to personal and interpersonal epistemology.

Social Exchange Theory

According to *social exchange theory,* social behavior in a given dyadic relationship is maintained by a high level of rewards relative to costs (Homans, 1958, 1974; Thibaut & Kelly, 1959). *Rewards* are defined as "pleasures, satisfactions, and gratifications the person enjoys," and *costs* are defined as "factors which operate to inhibit or deter the performance of a sequence of behavior" (Thibaut & Kelly, 1959, p. 12). Low reward exchange in the marital relationship can be anticipated to result in active consideration of alternative social exchanges perceived as potentially having higher levels of relative rewards to cost (comparison level of alternatives). It is assumed that each marital partner seeks to maximize rewards and minimize costs in the relationship.

In a given behavioral exchange, a partner emits a behavior that is received (labeled) by the mate as punishing or rewarding—or perhaps a combination of both properties. The mate emits a response that likewise may be received by the partner as punishing, rewarding, or both. The tendency of a partner to emit a behavior intended to elicit a sense of reward in the mate is assumed to be a product of (1) a history of high reward exchange, (2) an immediate sense of high reward in the relationship in the mind of the sender, and (3) a comparative appraisal of alternatives as being high in potential punishment and low in potential reward. The collective outcomes of ongoing exchanges determine the probability of a rewarding exchange, the level of satisfaction in the relationship, and the commitment to stay in the marriage.

It is important to note that a variety of cognitive processes are inherent in behavioral exchange, including perception, coding, appraisals, and attributions. The role of mediation in the ascription of meaning to a stimulus is profound in producing the ultimate valence and strength of the stimulus. The attached meaning fundamentally determines the impact of a spouse's behavior.

To summarize, Jacobson (1981) succinctly states that "a social learning model posits that the rate of reinforcers received from the partner determines not only the degree of subjective satisfaction but also the rate of rewards directed in return toward the partner. The principle that over time rewards given and received within a marital relationship are highly correlated is termed reciprocity, and by now numerous investigations have supported the lawfulness of this phenomenon in couples (p. 559).

Reciprocity

Reciprocity is defined as the tendency of couples to reward one another at approximately equal rates (Patterson & Reid, 1970). Each partner behaves in a manner to stimulate reinforcement consistent with his/her history of reinforcement and to satisfy the goal of equity. Jacobson and Margolin (1979) describe the processes of influence and control in a marital relationship as mutual, reciprocal, and circular.

Each action on the part of a mate is both a response to the partner's stimuli and a stimulus to the partner. Punctuating the interaction at any given point to identify singular cause is a violation of the process of interaction. With regard to distressed as opposed to nondistressed couples, reciprocity of positive exchanges is equally characteristic. However, reciprocity of punishing stimuli appears only characteristic of distressed couples (Birchler, 1973). Additionally, it has been found that all couples tend to produce highly correlated rates of rewarding and punishing exchanges on individually selected days (Wills, Weiss, & Patterson, 1974).

More recent explorations into the phenomenon of behavioral exchange conducted by Jacobson and his colleagues (1980, 1982) have exposed a difference in "reactivity" between distressed and nondistressed couples. Distressed couples have been found to be hypersensitive on a subjective, affective level to their partners' immediate behavior. Interpreting these findings, Jacobson (1984) states "that punishing behaviors have a negative impact on distressed couples not simply because they occur but because of the extreme

---

reaction that each spouse has to the partner's delivery of punishing behavior. Somehow, happy couples have devised a mechanism to neutralize the impact of negative behavior, and this mechanism is lacking in distressed couples (pp. 288–289).

Although there appears to be adequate support for the principle of reciprocity in couple interaction (Birchler, 1973; Gottman et al., 1976; Gottman, Markman, & Notarius, 1977; Jacobson, Waldron, & Moore, 1980; Patterson & Reid, 1970; Robinson & Price, 1980; Wills, Weiss, & Patterson, 1974), determining the specific expectations, desires, and obligations held by each partner to satisfy the goal of positive reciprocity is no small task. Sager (1976) identifies these factors as contractual terms that exist (1) only partially disclosed to the partner, (2) partially ill formed within the individual due to a lack of self-awareness, and (3) in a state of change as the marriage progresses, different stages of the life-cycle are attained and outside forces impinge on the couple individually or collectively. The anticipation of each partner that in exchange for what he or she will give to the other he or she will receive what that partner wants is predicated on each partner operating on a shared set of contractual terms. As noted above, a high level of awareness is typically not the case. Beyond awareness, of course, there must be agreement on the part of one mate with the other's terms and an ability to comply. Skill, knowledge, time, energy, and other resource deficiencies could all serve as barriers to a positive exchange.

Collaborative Set

Collaborative set is an acceptance on the part of each partner that they both have contributed to their discord and that effective change will require the effort of each of them. Inherent in this acceptance is acknowledgment of the interactional nature of marital functioning, that each has acted to influence and control the behavior of the other to promote the satisfaction of his/her own expectations and desires. Current distress is attributed to mutual behavioral excesses and deficits, mutual perceptual and information processing errors, and an overall failure to operate with shared contractual terms. It is incumbent upon the therapist to convince the couple of the advisability of viewing their relationship from the collaborative perspective. Jacobson and Margolin (1979) found that "if the therapist's theory, which emphasizes reciprocal causality and the necessity of mutual change, is sufficiently persuasive, couples might be convinced to alter their own theories, and thereby adopt the perspective of the therapist, from which will follow collaborative behavior" (p. 135).

Jacobson and Margolin (1979) **Assessment**
identified the purpose of assess-
ment as providing information that is necessary to (1) describe problems in the relationship, (2) identify variables that control the problem
behaviors, (3) select appropriate therapeutic interventions, and (4)
recognize when the intervention has been effective. A thorough
assessment needs to be comprehensive and specific, historic and contemporary, initial and ongoing, interactional and individual problem
oriented, and couple–relationship as well as therapy–process oriented.

The relative benefits of both comprehensive and specific assessment information can be realized as applied to marital satisfaction.
An overall satisfaction level may provide important global baseline
information while satisfaction with specific areas of marital functioning may expose strengths and weaknesses in the relationship. A comparison of specific satisfaction levels partner to partner may expose
significant disparity in subjective experience and expectancy.

Although a rationale can be built for the primary focus of assessment to address current cognitive and behavioral excesses and deficits
contributing to the couple's distress, gathering individual prerelation-
ship history and the couple's developmental history is advisable. It
is not uncommon that patterns of interaction characteristic of the couple have been played out over an extended period of time. Conditioned
patterns of interaction may continue even though the current reward
value of such behavior is minimal. Gaining an understanding of the
developmental bases of such phenomena as expectations, reinforcers,
behavior patterns, emotional episodes, and patterns of control may
provide valuable insight into the context of such phenomena, including
antecedent conditions and relationship-specific and extraneous controlling factors. Weiss (1984a) explains context as encompassing
history of interaction including cognitive and affective influences, actual competencies and resources available to the couple—"In a word,
'context' includes everything that the couple brings with them to the
interaction" (p. 233). Combining historic and current data may expose
repetitive, rather stable and static patterns of interaction. Haley (1976)
asserts that the discovery of repetitive sequences of behavior that
maintain dysfunctional behavior are potentially of greatest
significance to the therapist.

Although the predominant focus of assessment is on couple interaction, individual behavioral and emotional maladjustment and
psychopathology may be evident. Such maladjustment may have ex-
isted prior to the union or emerged after marriage. Hafner (1986) states
that "the emergence of psychological symptoms as a result of marital
interaction is by no means confined to marriages based on matching
psychopathology or overt maladjustment in one or both partners. It

may occur when seemingly well-adjusted people choose marriage partners in response to the competitive nature of modern society" (p. 69). Where individual maladjustment is evident, assessment methodologies tailored to both the individual and the couple should be introduced. For example, the treatment of a couple in which one partner is clinically depressed ideally would incorporate an assessment and intervention procedure sensitive both to the individual symptoms of depression as well as the role of depression in the couple's interaction. Couple interaction variables would include the behaviors of the nondepressed spouse that serve to stimulate and reinforce the depression, and the benefits the nondepressed spouse receives from his/her mate's depression.

In addition to the above, assessment of the couple's response to therapy and the therapist is important. This includes appraising the openness of the couple to express content and feelings in therapy, degree of assumption of collaborative set, willingness to complete homework, acceptance of the therapist's control of the therapy session, and tolerance for explanation, interpretation, and feedback. It also includes ongoing explication of goals and process of therapy and degree of client commitment to stated process and goals, as well as explication of evolving client-held expectations regarding the therapist's role.

Assessment methods include both conjoint and individual clinical interviews, self-report indexes and questionnaires, daily data collection measures and structured procedures to evaluate communication, problem solving, and information processing. Specific techniques and measures of data collection are described in numerous sources (Filsinger & Lewis, 1981; Jacobson, Elwood, & Dallas, 1981; Jacobson & Margolin, 1979; Kendall & Hollon, 1981; Margolin & Jacobson, 1981; Stuart, 1980; Weiss, 1984; Weiss & Margolin, 1977).

The initial assessment should be organized around several factors (Table 1).

Intervention

Engaging the couple in effective change can be a delicate process. Although it is important to be attentive to the specific expectations of the couple regarding the therapy process, goals in therapy and the therapist's role, it is the therapist's responsibility to take control and guide the couple in treatment. Inducting the couple into therapy requires a sensitivity to the emotions of each partner while gathering the information that comprises the initial assessment. At times, clients' demands for intervention conflict with the responsibility to complete the assessment adequately. The therapist may be required to "build

Table 1

Organizational Tools for Assessment

Satisfaction level (global and specific)
    communication
    conflict management
    sex
    finances
    support
    decision making
    trust
    affection
    household responsibilities
    time spent together
    time spent apart
    child management
What prompted the couple to seek therapy at this time
Presenting problem(s)—target behaviors
Early relationship attractions
Personal history
Client therapy goals
Commitment to staying married
Relationship developmental history
Information processing skills and errors
Thought disorders
Expectations
Communication patterns and properties
Relationship strengths—cognitive and behavioral skills relevant to coupling
Individual psychopathology
Environmental factors—stresses on the relationship (e.g., extended family interference)

a case" for data gathering and initially offer only minimal intervention input.

There are several responsibilities of the therapist in the application of C–BMT. The following procedures are significant in shaping the couple's expectations regarding the therapy process and in promoting the development of knowledge necessary to engage in effective treatment.

• *Fostering Collaborative Set.* The view that the marital problems are interactional; each partner has contributed knowingly and unintentionally to the distress; and that change on the part of both partners is required for effective outcomes.

• *Explanation of the Overall Goals of Therapy.* Somewhat variable, specifically dependent upon the status of the couple. For those who are fully committed to remaining married, the goal is to promote constructive change to: (1) reduce the frequency, intensity, and duration of conflict and unhappiness; (2) increase positively rewarding interchanges in the couple relationship; and (3) enhance the satisfaction level of each partner. For those couples who are contemplating divorce or are undecided, the goal is to interrupt dysfunctional marital interaction and to promote optimal functioning as a couple to facilitate decision making to either maintain the marriage or divorce. If the couple is separated, an altered intervention plan is required to meet the unique needs inherent in separation (Granvold, 1983; Granvold & Tarrant, 1983).

• *Explanation of the Assessment Process.* The therapist provides the couple with an understanding of the importance of developing a treatment plan based on a comprehensive yet specific understanding of the couple's functioning. The therapist sets the expectation with the couple that they participate actively in the assessment process (although it may be considered laborious and too time consuming at times) in order that a responsible treatment plan can be generated and evaluated for effectiveness.

• *Promote "Collaborative Empiricism."* Engaging the couple as participants and collaborators in formulating the treatment plan, a plan that "tests out" hypotheses regarding behavioral exchanges and relationship satisfaction; cognitive factors such as automatic thoughts, inferences, conclusions, and assumptions; and communication/problem-solving skills and relationship satisfaction. The concept of collaborative empiricism, introduced by Beck and his colleagues in their treatment of depression, calls on the therapist to be continuously active and deliberately interacting with the client(s), and to use ingenuity and resourcefulness to stimulate the active engagement of the client(s) in the therapeutic effort (Beck et al., 1979).

• *Promote Positive Expectancies.* The effort is to alter the typical negative-biased perspective of the couple and to instill confidence that the therapist can guide them in constructive change. With regard to negative bias, Jacobson and Margolin (1979) and Stuart (1975, 1980) suggest a focus on the strengths of the relationship and a sensitivity to positive spouse behavior as a means to dilute the negative bias. Beginning with the initial interview, the couple is encouraged to track the positives in the relationship. This focus on positive interchanges between spouses, both within sessions and between sessions, is emphasized throughout the course of treatment.

Presenting the professional credentials and experience of the therapist, reporting past success with couples in their change efforts, and therapist statement of confidence in his or her methods are useful methods to instill a sense of confidence in the therapist and a sense of optimism and hope regarding the benefits of the therapy process.

• *Explanation of the Complexity of Relationship Interaction.* The therapist explains the concept of social exchange theory as it relates

to the couple's relationship; the role of cognitive factors in human functioning and spouse interaction; learning theory as it relates to each
spouse and the change process; and behavioral excesses and deficits
relevant to marital interaction and therapeutic change.

• *Contracting.* The couple is asked to commit to a minimum of 8
weeks of marital treatment, meeting with the therapist conjointly approximately weekly (one-hour sessions) and one session each individually during the first three weeks. The couple is expected to continue
therapy as prescribed for the duration of the eight weeks, to take no
definitive legal action to dissolve the marriage during the time commitment, and, consistent with Stuart's (1975) long-standing recommen-
dation, to act "as if" the marriage is successful and will be maintained.
The latter contract term is particularly important in shaping the couple's expectations and perceptions. At the end of the 8-week time
period, the course of treatment will be evaluated, and, if therapy is
continued, new treatment goals and time parameters will be defined.
If termination takes place at that time, follow-up and relevant subsequent individual treatment should be scheduled.

• *Homework.* The couple is informed that specific homework
assignments will be made at each session and reviewed at the subsequent session. These assignments may be oriented to assessment or
change, individual or couple, cognitive or behavioral, shared or
private, and specifically defined or general for the purpose of promoting novelty and ingenuity.

The specific techniques of C–BMT can be organized under four
major headings: behavior exchange, communication training, problem
solving, and cognitive–behavioral intervention. Each intervention
methodology has a relevant role to fulfill in the comprehensive treatment of marital discord. The author's approach to marital therapy
relies heavily on each methodology. BMT methods are well established and are presented clearly and comprehensively in many sources
(for example, Bornstein & Bornstein, 1986; Jacobson, 1981; Jacobson & Margolin, 1979; O'Leary & Turkewitz, 1978; Stuart, 1980;
Weiss, 1978). However, the application of cognitive approaches to the
treatment of marital problems has only begun to emerge. It is for these
reasons that the remainder of this article focuses only on cognitive intervention strategies as applied to marital discord.

Cognitive factors play a significant role   **C–BMT**
in marital interaction in many ways.
Behavior on the part of one spouse is mediated by the other in terms
of meaning, motivation, and etiology. A variety of cognitive distortions and thinking errors can be identified that could account, in part,

for marital distress. Expectations regarding "appropriate," desirable, and necessary behavior reside privately within each spouse and are applied to appraise interaction and serve as a mechanism for the subjective determination of happiness and marital satisfaction. These appraisals take place situationally and also accumulate to form overall contentment and shape the evolution of expectations regarding one's own behavior, spouse's behavior, and marriage per se.

Belief systems and attitudes about self are important particularly regarding an individual's appraisal of the comparison level of alternatives. If the spouse holds the traditional belief in the intrinsic permanence of marriage, that it is a lifelong contract, binding on both partners, that should not be dissolved no matter how punishing the situation, the spouse may be inclined to stay in the marriage despite low rewards (Scanzoni, 1972). Or perhaps his or her commitment to remain in a distressed relationship can be traced to the perception of himself or herself as incapable of successfully detaching from the spouse, adjusting to single life and living independently. Several conceptualizations have been developed to account for an individual's sense of competency to act on his or her world (execute a certain behavior pattern) including self-efficacy (Bandura, 1977, 1978a, 1978b; Weiss, 1984b), learned helplessness (Seligman, 1975), and locus of control (Rotter, 1966). The cognitive mechanisms influencing an individual to remain in a relationship predominated by a schedule of low rewards and substantial punishment require much further exploration.

The assumption of continuity between overt and covert learning principles (Mahoney, 1974) is critically important in the application of internal mediational processes to the analysis and treatment of marital distress. In essence, private events are considered to be subject to conditioning. "Thoughts, images, memories, and sensations are described as covert stimuli, covert responses, or covert consequences . . . subject to reinforcement, punishment, and extinction" (p. 61). Extrapolating from this position, it is feasible that covert behavior chains are conditioned and became applied actively in the regulation of interpersonal interaction. This is not to say that these processes function independently from an external environment, but rather, form one component of the interaction between external and internal stimuli in promoting behavior. However, covert conditioning may be accountable for a negative behavior exchange between a couple in which overt behavioral factors would appear to clearly promote a positive exchange. To illustrate, an individual who has become conditioned to a high rate of punishment throughout his life before marriage may behave to sabotage rewarding interaction as a means of promoting the schedule of punishment consistent with his conditioning.

Such behavior may defy the principle of reciprocity in which positive is exchanged for positive. The interaction may be punctuated as rewarding behavior from wife to husband (experienced and labeled as rewarding by the husband), followed by the husband's punishing behavior toward the wife (experienced and labeled as punishing by the wife), followed by punishing behavior from the wife toward her husband (intended as punishing by the wife and experienced as punishing by the husband). Although this behavioral exchange appears illogical, the assumption is that it satisfies a hidden agenda that may have little rational connection with the current situation.

The challenge confronting the cognitive–behavioral marital therapist is to expose those mediational factors that serve to promote marital distress and dissatisfaction and to effect change in and through those processes. In support of this challenge, Jacobson (1984) specified three ways in which dysfunctional cognitive processes can subvert the process of change in BMT: (1) cognitive and perceptual processes can remain dysfunctional, despite successfully induced behavior change; (2) dysfunctional cognitive and perceptual processes can interfere with the behavior change itself, such that spouses will avoid complying with therapeutic directives or in other ways refuse to enact positive behavior changes; and (3) dysfunctional cognitive and perceptual processes can become functionally autonomous from any behavioral referent (p. 287). It is apparent that a "marriage" of cognitive and behavioral methods may prove efficacious in treating marital distress.

Faulty Information Processing

One level of intervention in C–BMT is the information processing component of functioning. The following are cognitive distortions common to information processing.

Absolutistic, Dichotomous Thinking

The tendency to view experiences, objects, and situations in a polarized manner: good/bad, right/wrong, strong/weak. Mary, upset with her husband, John, for failing to assert himself in collecting the delinquent rent payment from the renters, refers to John as a "spineless, weak man." John likewise views himself as spineless and weak. When John and Mary enter marital treatment their verbal conflict rate is daily. Later in therapy, after a reduction to approximately one conflict per 10 days, John and Mary enter the session stating that the marriage is "no good" because they had a disagreement. Absolustic thinking simplifies and distorts the meaning of life events. It is illogical because a given condition or experience rarely can be rated objectively as one extreme or another. While the client might subjectively feel totally bad about an experience or currently be making an absolutistic judgment about it, he or she may be instructed in the wisdom of alternative feelings and views.

Overgeneralization

Refers to the pattern of drawing a general rule or conclusion on the basis of one or more isolated incidents and applying the concept across the board to related and unrelated situations (Beck et al., 1979). Susie is typically not sexually provocative. One evening she dons a skimpy negligee and her husband, Joe, who is usually attentive to her, responds in an otherwise preoccupied, inattentive, and sexually disinterested manner. Susie thinks, "I can't turn Joe on; I'm just not a lover. I'm not going to wear any more sexy clothes because it just doesn't work."

Selective Abstraction

Typically is a focus on the negative in a situation, ignoring other positive (sometimes more salient) features and viewing the entire experience as negative based upon the selective view. For example, Bart and Jane are at Jane's company cocktail party. They are attentive to one another throughout the evening. Jane's boss, Arlene, asks to speak with Jane privately for 15 minutes, during which time Bart is left to socialize on his own. Lacking well-developed social skills, Bart feels insecure and awkward while Jane is away. Upon her return, Bart acts coldly toward Jane and asks to leave the party immediately. Bart thinks, "this whole night has been unpleasant," and states to Jane, "I really don't appreciate being left alone all night." Bart overlooked the fact that the part of the evening before Jane went with her boss had been pleasant and that Jane had only left for 15 minutes of the three hours they attended the party.

Arbitrary Inference

Reaching an arbitrary negative conclusion when there is no evidence to support the conclusion or there is evidence to the contrary. Freeman (1983) describes two types of arbitrary inference as mind reading and negative prediction:

1. Mind Reading. Cathy and Paul had tentatively agreed to eat dinner together after Paul's golf game. When Paul called home to say he was on his way Cathy said, "I'm not going to eat but I'll put a steak

on for you." Paul angrily responded, "I'm not coming home to eat alone; you would rather watch TV than eat with me anyway." To further illustrate, Bob asks Nancy, "Where are you going?" Nancy thinks, "Bob is trying to control me." Mind reading may also relate to feelings. "You're mad, I can tell because you didn't kiss me when you came home."

2. Negative Prediction. This type of arbitrary inference involves imagining or anticipating something bad or unpleasant is going to happen without adequate or realistic support for the prediction. A functionally orgasmic woman has failed to reach an orgasm during the past four sexual encounters with her husband (each encounter experienced while she was very fatigued). The woman states, "I'm never going to have an orgasm again; when you lose it (the ability), it's gone forever." She becomes disinterested in sexual contact with her mate, and becomes cold and aloof.

Magnification and Minimization

Errors in evaluating the significance or magnitude of a behavior, condition or event that are so extreme as to constitute a distortion. Imperfections in oneself and others are magnified, while talents, knowledge, and skill are minimized. Magnification may result in becoming extremely emotional and critical over the misdeeds or human errors of others. Ann forgot to take the dog to the veterinarian for an unscheduled routine vaccination visit. When Del was informed he became extremely angry and chastising of Ann. Perceptual blinders may serve to filter the meaning of one's own and others' talents, positive qualities, and performances. After 12 years with the firm, Mary Ann became one of the 15 percent to become a partner. She believes and states that, "anyone could have done it."

Personalization

The act of relating a negative event or situation to oneself without the adequate causal evidence to make the connection. This is a form of attribution, a process which will receive more attention later. There are two forms of personalization. In the first instance an arbitrary conclusion is reached in which a negative event is viewed as caused by the subject. To illustrate, Larry didn't eat lunch because his wife failed to put his lunch by his briefcase that morning. Linda thought, "I'm responsible for Larry missing lunch" (although Larry could either have eaten out or remembered the lunch even though it was not in its usual place by his briefcase). Linda further thought of herself as an uncaring wife for her action. In the second form of personalization, an arbitrary conclusion is reached in which one views himself or herself as the object of a negative event, and therefore causally connected. Kay encounters a traffic jam on the way to meet Roger for lunch and concludes, "If I didn't have a lunch date with Roger, there wouldn't be a traffic jam!" Kay failed to allow adequate time for the typical heavy midday traffic.

The view that a given behavior is produced out of a negative motivation.
Mahoney (1974) defines *attribution* as im-

**Negative
Attribution**

plied causality. Attributions often are simplistic statements that are perceived as accountable for a given behavior. The tendency is to attribute singular causation to complex patterns of behavior. Negative attributions can take the form of blaming, "you make me so mad," in which the responsibility for the anger is displaced to the mate. Hurvitz (1975) presents a form of negative attributions as "terminal hypotheses" in which behavior, meanings, or feelings are interpreted such that change cannot take place. Included are such determinants of behavior as psychological classifications ("You're a manic depressive"); pseudoscientific labels ("You're a Virgo, that's why you act the way you do"); and inappropriate generalizations about innate qualities or traits that cannot be changed ("He has no will power, was born that way; that's why he's so fat"). Epstein (1982) identifies behavior changes that are attributed to coercion or impression management: "He's doing more chores around the house because he's afraid I'll leave him if he doesn't." This form of attribution frequently is centered around therapist-assigned behaviors: "You're only being nice to me because the therapist told you to be more pleasant." The implication is that the only reason behind such behavior is the assignment and that being more pleasant is actually misrepresentative of the spouse's desires. Another form of negative attribution is malevolent intent: "You purposefully came home late to make me worry about you." "You took your secretary to lunch to make me jealous." Another negative attribution has ingredients of mind reading and inferential reasoning associated with it: "If you loved me you'd know what I want from you right now." The fact that he is not doing what she "wants" is, by her inference, motivated by a lack of love—presumably considered a negative by her. To restate the attribution, "Your lack of love for me is causing you to be insensitive to what I want from you at this moment." Such a thought pattern also qualifies as an unrealistic expectation.

The interpretation of a message incon- **Faulty**
sistent with the intention; a discrepancy be- **Interpretation**
tween intent and impact (Gottman, 1979).
Louis made the following statement about his colleague at work: "I
don't care much for Arthur." (Louis' intention was only to share his
feeling regarding Arthur with his wife). His wife, Arlene, thinks,
"Louis doesn't like his job." Such an interpretation may go unvalidated
and give rise to an emotive and possibly overt behavioral response
followed by a stream of evaluative, interpretive, and problem-solving,
action-oriented thoughts. This covert activity may be largely accountable for the subsequent behavior. Arlene became physically tense and
said, "I wish we hadn't bought this house and taken on such a high
house payment." Her thought process flowed from "Louis doesn't like
his job," to "He may quit or take another job, perhaps for less money,"
to "If he does that I'm worried that we won't be able to make the house
payment." Arlene's concomitant emotional response was anxiety,
coupled with some mounting hostility toward Louis over his putting
them in such a financial bind (were he to act in accordance with her
chain of thoughts). Louis, of course, is unaware of Arlene's chain of
thoughts (unless she verbalizes them) and covertly responds with
curiosity regarding the connection between his comment about Arthur and Arlene's comment about the purchase of their house. In sum,
the discrepancy between intent and impact is the product of a faulty
interpretation followed by an invalidated stream of thought.

The procedure common to the treatment of all information processing errors involves identification of adequate, logical evidence to support
the conclusions. It is for this reason that the process of "collaborative
empiricism" is so important. As the couple and therapist generate possible hypotheses related to the interactional conclusions reached, the il-
logic in the thinking will surface with deliberate and focused guidance
from the therapist, the initial lack of awareness of the self-sustained
cognitive distortions and the emotional overlay associated with such
thinking will evolve into the client's organized evaluation of the validi-
ty of the hypotheses that have heretofore operated automatically, in-
validly in his or her thinking. As a result, change can be expected in
the spouse's view of self, of partner, and in the negative emotional
episodes that have punctuated the couple's interaction.

The cognitive distortions identified in **Irrational Be-**
the preceding discussion may exist rather **liefs and Faulty**
harmlessly at a low rate of performance in **Expectations**
the nondistressed individual. Or perhaps, an
individual may be subject to "pocket" distortions, which contribute to

problematical marital interaction but exist as exceptions to typically logical thinking. Intervention focused on "blind spots" in the spouse's thought processes may produce relatively rapid change. In cases where the distortions are severe, extensive, and intractable, however, treatment requires an exploration of the individual's personal philosophy. Cognitive distortions emerge from and are governed by an underlying set of rules including such elements as cognitive organization, structural causal theories, attitudes toward oneself and toward reality, and belief system. Terminology used to identify an individual's underlying set of rules varies as follows: personal constructs (Kelly, 1955); irrational beliefs (Ellis, 1973, 1977); automatic thoughts and schemas (Beck, 1976; Beck et al., 1979); and paradigm (Guidano & Liotti, 1983). The term *irrational beliefs* is used here as representative of a personal philosophy that promotes a distortion in thought processes and leads to emotional, behavioral, and interpersonal dysfunction.

There have been several initial efforts made to apply cognitive restructuring methods to the treatment of marital distress (Abrahms, 1983; Bedrosian, 1983; Ellis, 1969, 1977; Epstein, 1982; Epstein & Eidelson, 1981; Jacobson, 1984; Jacobson & Holtzworth-Munroe, 1986; McClellan & Stieper, 1977; Revenstorf, 1984; Schindler & Vollmer, 1984; Weiss, 1984b). Common among the procedures outlined by these authors is the identification of unrealistic, demanding expectations of self and the marital partner, specification of faulty attributions, and a deliberate effort on the part of the therapist to foster the clients' disengagement from maladaptive beliefs and judgments. While listening to clients speak, the therapist listens for evidence of their causal theories, basic assumptions, or irrational beliefs. These are framed as hypotheses and collaboratively the therapist and couple proceed to disprove or confirm them through logical, empirical challenge.

Ellis (1962) has identified 11 irrational beliefs that serve as the basis for dysfunctional thinking and faulty expectations. These beliefs incorporate such imperatives as (1) the demand (as opposed to the desire) for love and approval, perfection, and control over one's world; (2) freedom from self-responsibility for one's own emotions; (3) extreme dependency on others; (4) an irrefutable right to blame others for one's own and others' imperfections and shortcomings; and (5) the indelible effect of history on current behavior and emotions. Only a few irrational beliefs are identified and discussed as they relate to marital distress.

Demanding Love, Attention, and Approval

It is not uncommon for the marital partner to fix his or her identity in the marital relationship to the extent that the continuation of the marriage is imperative for a sense of "ok-ness" as a human being. Thoughts such as "I would be nothing without you," and "I can't stand the thought of losing you" promote potential dysfunction. The demand for continued partnership and approval may result in the subordination of one mate to the other. Intolerance of criticism, disagreement, and conflict may be based on approval needs. Feelings of hurt and overwhelming thoughts of self-loathing result. Extreme anxiety, fear, depression, and worry may exist in anticipation of disapproval or abandonment. If unchanged, these rather unappealing emotions may actually promote the feared outcome. The spouse with strong approval needs and low self-regard is likely to view a mate's criticism of him or her as based on fact and unbiased observation, processed in a flawless mind. The deferential spouse places complete credence in his or her mate's observations, and is therefore unmotivated to seek substantiating evidence or in any way challenge the mate.

Alternatively, demands for love and approval may exist along with insensitive, disrespectful, or untoward behavior. The spouse expects noncontingent acceptance of his or her behavior on the basis of human rights and a distorted view of spouse obligation and duty. Rigid expectations of devotion and compliance with idiosyncratic wishes emerge from egocentrism and hedonism. Noncompliance with rigid, intractable expectations of unconditional acceptance results in emotional coercion in the form of anger, depression, coldness, rejection, and other means of "retaliatory" punishment.

Other specific behavioral expectations are implicit, requiring inferential determination. An individual with strong approval needs may go to great lengths to comply with inferred expectations, with a reciprocal expectation of love and approval to confirm the accuracy of the inferences made. A series of trial-and-error exercises may proceed in search of the proper match between expectation and performance. If the independent spouse's expectations are capricious, the dependent spouse's approval needs may be satisfied at a low and apparently random rate. In this manner, the independent spouse can maintain control over his or her partner through the manipulation of approval needs. If the reinforcement rate is low and apparently random as experienced by the dependent spouse, the likely outcome over time is marital unhappiness and/or individual disturbance (e.g., passivity or apathy depression).

Things Must Go My Way

Demandingness; excessive control over oneself, others, and the world; and narcissism are the elements of this irrational belief. The demanding spouse informs his or her mate of unmet or marginally satisfied expectations through anger, anxiety, resentment, worry, depression, hostility, or preoccupation with himself. The expectation is that the mate views the world exactly as he or she does—has the same interests, tastes, desires, and beliefs. Differences and conflict are not tolerated passively and are viewed as threats to sense of self and in violation of a fixed view of marriage. When differences are verbalized or show up in behavior, a strong emotional response is likely along with a corresponding behavioral manisfestation. Low frustration tolerance predominates. Rules of family functioning and couple interaction must coincide with expectations: "I can't stand it when you're late." "A married person is not supposed to be attached to anyone other than the spouse." The spouse expects to be in control of his or her mate and world as much as is possible. The spouse may truly believe that is it better to control his or her mate because he or she can do such a better job of it. The spouse is highly prone to catastrophising when the mate or significant other violates or challenges him or her, or that expectations of the world are violated. He or she has little tolerance for the exigencies of life.

The belief results in blaming and plac-   *It's Your Fault*
ing responsibility for one's own emotions
external to oneself. The spouse holds the mate responsible for happiness/unhappiness and uses emotional coercion to shape the mate's behavior. The spouse seldom accepts responsibility for his or her own behavior. He or she is intolerant of the mate's error-proneness and calls names and labels the mate. Any wrongdoing for which the spouse is responsible is viewed as absolutely in response to what the mate did *first*. Current predicaments and problems are viewed as the product of the mate's wrongdoing or poor judgment. Any acceptance of wrongdoing is viewed as documentation of not "ok-ness" and, hence, he or she is well defended against it. His or her defensive, negative thinking pattern over a prolonged period typically renders him or her pessimistic and possessed of a dim view of self, his or her mate, world, and future. As a consequence, the spouse tends to expect negatives and seemingly delights in sharing negative expectations with his or her mate.

The following interaction is illustrative of various information processing errors, cognitive distortions, and exaggerated expectations that can punctuate a distressed couple's interaction (H = husband, W = wife):

H: I knew that the house would look like s--- when I got home even though you had the day off [negative expectation]. You ran around town spending money and visiting your friends...any excuse not to clean the place up [negative attribution].

W: You think I'm on this earth to please you...that I'm your slave [mind reading]. If you'd help out once in a while...[blaming].

H: I do help out...who do you think supports this family [cognitive distortion]? You are screwed up in the head, Wanda [terminal hypothesis/labeling].

W: Hank [*Wanda escalates her voice volume and flushes; appears angry*] you disgust me [blaming]...throwing up to me your money! What about the money *I* make? Oh, what the hell...I want to tell you something about the house. You expect it to be perfect, flawless [mind reading]. We don't live in a vacuum. I think the house is good enough, given the kids and our schedules [rational statement of values and expectations].

H: There you go again with that same old excuse—the kids [negative perception]. They were your idea anyway [blaming]!

W: You're just like your father [terminal hypothesis]! He doesn't give a s--- about you and you don't give a s--- about the kids [mind reading/dichotomous thinking]!

H: I do too, it's just that....

W: It's just that they're not perfect. You and your perfectionism [mind reading/labeling/terminal hypothesis].

H: The kids never mind a thing that is said to them [total/absolutistic thinking]. And you don't ever hold them accountable for their chores [total/absolutistic thinking].

W: Kids aren't *supposed* to have to do the dishes all the time. They're supposed to be able to be kids [realistic expectations].

H: Kids are to be held accountable for their chores and that's it...[demandingness]. You marshmallow [labeling/terminal hypothesis].

W: What do you mean by that?

H: You're a marshmallow, that's that [labeling/terminal hypothesis]!

W: Well, you're a jerk...and that's that [retaliatory labeling]!

C–BMT Needs Validation

The evidence that cognitive methods have been efficacious in the treatment of other problems promotes a sense of optimism regarding their application to marital problems. The challenge confronting the C–BMT clinician–researcher is to validate empirically the methods employed, and, in so doing, guide the expansion of cognitive strategies for use in marital treatment and refine those procedures found to be effective.

Abrahms, J. L. (1983). Cognitive–behavioral strategies to induce and enhance a collaborative set in distressed couples. In A. Freeman (Ed.), *Cognitive therapy with couples and groups* (pp. 125–155). New York: Plenum.

Bandura, A. (1977). Self-efficacy: Toward a unifying theory of behavior change. *Psychological Review, 84,* 191–215.

Bandura, A. (1978a). Reflections on self-efficacy. *Advances in Behaviour Research and Therapy, 1,* 237–269.

Bandura, A. (1978b). The self system in reciprocal determinism. *American Psychologist, 33,* 344–358.

Beck, A. T. (1976). *Cognitive therapy and the emotional disorders.* New York: International Universities.

Beck, A. T., Rush, A. J., Shaw, B. F., & Emery, G. (1979). *Cognitive therapy of depression.* New York: Guilford.

Bedrosian, R. C. (1983). Cognitive therapy in the family system. In A. Freeman (Ed.), *Cognitive therapy with couples and groups* (pp. 95–106). New York: Plenum.

Birchler, G. R. (1973). Differential patterns of instrumental affiliative behavior as a function of degree of marital distress and level of intimacy. *Dissertation Abstracts International, 33,* 14499B–4500B. (University Microfilms No. 73-7865, 102).

Bornstein, P. H., & Bornstein, M. T. (1986). *Marital therapy: A behavioral–communications approach.* New York: Pergamon.

Ellis, A. (1962). *Reason and emotion in psychotherapy.* New York: Lyle Stuart.

Ellis, A. (1969). Neurotic interaction between marital partners. In B. N. Ard & C. C. Ard (Eds.), *Handbook of marriage counseling* (pp. 367–373). Palo Alto, CA: Science and Behavior Books.

Ellis, A. (1973). *Humanistic psychotherapy.* New York: McGraw-Hill.

Ellis, A. (1977a). The basic clinical theory of rational–emotive therapy. In A. Ellis & R. Grieger, *Handbook of rational–emotive therapy* (pp. 3–34). New York: Springer.

Ellis, A. (1977b). The nature of disturbed marital interactions. In A. Ellis & R. Grieger, *Handbook of rational–emotive therapy* (pp. 170–176). New York: Springer.

Emery, H., Hollon, S. D., & Bedrosian, R. C. (Eds.). (1981). *New directions in cognitive therapy.* New York: Guilford.

Epstein, N. (1982). Cognitive therapy with couples. *The American Journal of Family Therapy, 10,* 5–16.

Epstein, N., & Eidelson, R. J. (1981). Unrealistic beliefs of clinical couples: Their relationship to expectations, goals, and satisfaction. *The American Journal of Family Therapy, 9,* 13–22.

Filsinger, E. E., & Lewis, R. A. (Eds.). (1981). *Assessing marriage: New behavioral approaches.* Beverly Hills, CA: Sage.

Freeman, A. (1983). Cognitive therapy: An overview. In A. Freeman (Ed.), *Cognitive therapy with couples and groups* (pp. 1–9). New York: Plenum.

Gottman, J., Markman, H., & Notarius, C. (1977). The topography of marital conflict: A sequential analysis of verbal and nonverbal behavior. *Journal of Marriage and the Family, 39,* 461–477.

Gottman, J., Notarius, C., Markman, H., Bank, S., Yoppi, B., & Rubin, M. E. (1976). Behavior exchange theory and marital decision making. *Journal of Personality and Social Psychology, 34,* 14–23.

Gottman, J. M. (1979). *Marital interaction.* New York: Academic.

Granvold, D. K. (1983). Structured separation for marital treatment and decision-making. *Journal of Marital and Family Therapy, 9,* 403–412.

Granvold, D. K., & Tarrant, R. (1983). Structured marital separation as a marital treatment method. *Journal of Marital & Family Therapy, 9,* 189–198.

Guidano, V. F., & Liotti, G. (1983). *Cognitive processes and emotional disorders.* New York: Guilford.

Hafner, R. J. (1986). *Marriage and mental illness: A sex-roles perspective.* New York: Guilford.

Haley, J. (1976). *Problem-solving therapy: New strategies for effective family therapy.* San Francisco: Jossey-Bass.

Hawkins, R. C., Fremouw, W. J., & Clement, P. F. (Eds.). (1984). *The binge–purge syndrome: Diagnosis, treatment, and research.* New York: Springer.

Homans, G. C. (1958). Social behavior as exchange. *American Journal of Sociology, 62,* 597–606.

Homans, G. C. (1974). *Social behavior: Its elementary forms.* New York: Harcourt, Brace & Jovanovich.

Hurvitz, N. (1975). Interaction hypotheses in marriage counseling. In A. S. Gurman & D. G. Rice (Eds.), *Couples in conflict* (pp. 225–240). New York: Aronson.

Jacobson, N. S. (1984). The modification of cognitive processes in behavioral marital therapy: Integrating cognitive and behavioral intervention strategies. In K. Hahlweg & N. S. Jacobson (Eds.), *Marital interaction* (pp. 285–308). New York: Guilford.

Jacobson, N. S., & Margolin, G. (1979). *Marital therapy: Strategies based on social learning and behavior exchange principles.* New York: Brunner/Mazel.

Jacobson, N. S., Waldron, H., & Moore, D. (1980). Toward a behavioral profile of marital distress. *Journal of Consulting & Clinical Psychology, 48,* 696–703.

Jacobson, N. S. (1981). Behavioral marital therapy. In A. S. Gurman & D. P. Kniskern (Eds.), *Handbook of family therapy* (pp. 556–591). New York: Brunner/Mazel.

Jacobson, N. S., Elwood, R., & Dallas, M. (1981). Assessment of marital dysfunction. In D. H. Barlow (Ed.), *Behavioral assessment of adult disorders* (pp. 439–479). New York: Guilford Press.

Jacobson, N. S., Follette, W. C., & McDonald, D. W. (1982). Reactivity to positive and negative behavior in distressed and nondistressed married couples. *Journal of Consulting & Clinical Psychology, 50,* 706–714.

Jacobson, N. S., & Holtzworth-Munroe, A. (1986). Marital therapy: A social learning–cognitive perspective. In N. S. Jacobson & A. S. Gurman (Eds.), *Clinical handbook of marital therapy* (pp. 29–70). New York: Guilford.

Kelly, G. (1955). *The psychology of personal constructs* (Vols. 1 & 2). New

York: Norton.

Kendall, P. C., & Hollon, S. D. (Eds.). (1981). *Assessment strategies for cognitive–behavioral interventions.* New York: Academic Press.

Liberman, R. (1975). Behavioral principles in family and couple therapy. In A. S. Gurman & D. G. Rice (Eds.), *Couples in conflict* (pp. 209–224). New York: Aronson.

Mahoney, M. J. (1974). *Cognition and behavior modification.* Cambridge, MA: Ballinger.

Margolin, G., & Jacobson, N. S. (1981). Assessment of marital dysfunction. In M. Hersen & A. S. Bellack (Eds.), *Behavioral assessment: A practical handbook* (2nd ed.; pp. 389–426). London: Pergamon.

McClellan, T. A., & Stieper, D. R. (1977). A structured approach to group marriage counseling. In A. Ellis & R. Grieger, *Handbook of rational–emotive therapy* (pp. 281–291). New York: Springer.

Meichenbaum, D. (1977). *Cognitive–behavior modification: An integrative approach.* New York: Plenum.

Michelson, L., & Ascher, L. M. (Eds.). (1987). *Anxiety and stress disorders: Cognitive–behavioral assessment and treatment.* New York: Guilford.

Novaco, R. W. (1975). *Anger control: The development and evaluation of an experimental treatment.* Lexington, MA: Lexington.

O'Leary, K. D., & Turkewitz, H. (1978). Marital therapy from a behavioral perspective. In T. J. Paolino & B. S. McCrady (Eds.), *Marriage and marital therapy: Psychoanalytic, behavioral and systems theory perspectives* (pp. 240–297). New York: Brunner/Mazel.

Patterson, G. R., & Reid, J. B. (1970). Reciprocity and coercion: Two facets of social systems. In C. Neuringer & J. C. Michael (Eds.), *Behavior modification in clinical psychology* (pp. 133–177). New York: Appleton–Century–Crofts.

Rappaport, A. F., & Harrel, J. E. (1975). *A behavioral exchange model for marital counseling.* In A. S. Gurman & D. G. Rice (Eds.), *Couples in conflict* (pp. 258–277). New York: Aronson.

Revenstorf, D. (1984). The role of attribution of marital distress in therapy. In K. Hahlweg & N. S. Jacobson (Eds.), *Marital interaction* (pp. 325–336). New York: Guilford.

Robinson, E. A., & Price, M. G. (1980). Pleasurable behavior in marital interaction: An observational study. *Journal of Consulting & Clinical Psychology, 48,* 117–118.

Rotter, J. B. (1966). Generalized expectancies for internal versus external control of reinforcement. *Psychological Monographs, 80,* (1, whole No. 609).

Sager, C. J. (1976). *Marriage contracts and couple therapy.* New York: Brunner/Mazel.

Scanzoni, J. (1972). *Sexual bargaining.* Englewood Cliffs, NJ: Prentice-Hall.

Schindler, L., & Vollmer, M. (1984). Cognitive perspectives in behavioral marital therapy: Some proposals for bridging theory, research, and practice. In K. Hahlweg & N. S. Jacobson (Eds.), *Marital interaction* (pp. 309–324). New York: Guilford.

Seligman, M.E.P. (1975). *Helplessness: On depression, development, and death.* San Francisco: Freeman.

Stuart, R. B. (1975). Behavioral remedies for marital ills: A guide to the use of operant–interpersonal techniques. In A. S. Gurman & D. G. Rice (Eds.), *Couples in conflict* (pp. 241–257). New York: Aronson.

Stuart, R. B. (1980). *Helping couples change: A social learning approach to marital therapy.* New York: Guilford.

Thibaut, J. W., & Kelly, H. H. (1959). *The social psychology of groups.* New York: Wiley.

Weiss, R. L. (1978). The conceptualization of marriage from a behavioral perspective. In T. J. Paolino & B. S. McCrady (Eds.), *Marriage and marital therapy: Psychoanalytic, behavioral and systems theory perspectives* (pp. 165–239). New York: Brunner/Mazel.

Weiss, R. L. (1984a). Cognitive and behavioral measures of marital interaction. In K. Hahlweg & N. S. Jacobson (Eds.), *Marital interaction: Analysis and modification* (pp. 232–252). New York: Guilford.

Weiss, R. L. (1984b). Cognitive and strategic interventions in behavioral marital therapy. In K. Hahlweg & N. S. Jacobson (Eds.), *Marital interaction: Analysis and modification* (pp. 337–355). New York: Guilford.

Weiss, R. L., & Margolin, G. (1977). Assessment of marital conflict and accord. In A. R. Ciminero, K. D. Calhoun, & H. E. Adams (Eds.), *Handbook of behavioral assessment* (pp. 555–602). New York: Wiley.

Wills, T. A., Weiss, R. L., & Patterson, G. R. (1974). A behavioral analysis of the determinants of marital satisfaction. *Journal of Consulting & Clinical Psychology, 42,* 802–811.

HEALING THE TRAUMA:
Treatment for Adult Survivors of Sexual Abuse
Brenda Wiewel

S exual abuse of children has come out of the bedroom into public media focus during the 1980s. The increased visibility allows many adult survivors to discuss how they were affected by their incest experience during the era before heightened public awareness. The understanding they needed from persons in helping professions was rarely available. One adult client reported that no one at school ever questioned her about her bruises, nervousness, or withdrawal. Professionally, it is the task of social workers to help ease the trauma for survivors who lived under the shadow of a secret no one seemed able to hear. Ideas on organizing common treatment themes in useful ways are presented in this article. A group format designed for survivors with major mental illness is discussed. Although one study (Rosenfeld, 1979) found that 33 percent of the psychiatric patients in the sample had an incest history, there is little written about how to adapt treatment strategies for these survivors.

Assessment of the impact of incest is an important part of treatment. Often survivors have other severe problems in addition to incest and do not connect their current concerns to their incest history (Courtois & Watts, 1982; Ellenson, 1985; Gelinas, 1983). Once the incest history has been elicited by a sensitive psychiatric examination, a clinician may want to predict which experiences will lead to the most severe trauma. However, the research shows that conclusions based on type of experience are not possible. Impact must be assessed on an individual basis (Courtois & Watts, 1982; Vander Mey & Neff, 1982). This concurs with another experience where one survivor who was fondled on her breasts by a stepfather had a severe reaction, including hallucinations of being touched on her breasts as an adult while reading, a chronic eating disorder, and inability to function sexually with her husband. Another survivor who had been sexually abused severely by her mother and her mother's male relatives reacted less severely with mild depression, emotional release upon recovering memories, and difficulty with self-assertion.

Common treatment themes can be organized into a sequential set of stages. The concept and content of the stages was developed initially by the author with the help and input of a colleague, Hal Platts, LCSW, at the Los Angeles County Mental Health Outpatient Clinic. These stages can be used in assessment of how a client is dealing with his or her incest history and as a direction for treatment efforts. The approach presented here parallels the work of major psychological theorists Erik Erikson and Elisabeth Kübler-Ross regarding "normal" human reactions to major life events. Erikson talked of developmental stages and tasks corresponding to different phases of the life-cycle (Erikson, 1963). Kübler-Ross identified sequential stages she thought to be experienced normally by dying patients and the therapeutic tasks necessary to move from one stage to another (Kübler-Ross, 1969). Teaching survivors about the normative stages allows them to gain perspective on their reactions and be prepared for what they may experience in the future.

The following discussion is based on a definition of incest, as cited in Benward and Densen-Ger- **Definition and Assumptions** ber (1975): "Sexual contact with a person who would be considered an ineligible partner because of his blood and/or social ties (that is, kin) to the subject and her family . . . the 'partner' represents someone from whom the child should rightfully expect warmth or protection and sexual distance" (p. 324). Courtois and Watts (1982) recommend that any definition should include an emphasis on "incest as sexual assault, especially in those cases where it was (a) coercive and nonconsensual, and (b) in cases involving cross-generational contact" (p. 277). The concepts presented here have been used with survivors in dealing with perpetrators of either sex.

An important underlying assumption of this mode of treatment is that incest may create trauma that *can* be resolved and may damage interpersonal skills that *can* be repaired. The damage stems from the survivor's experience with an authority figure who "knew what was best for her/him" and was "in control" over what happened. The aggressor was in control because she/he had the power to hurt or help the victim. The victim was controlled by his/her guilt, fear, and desire for attention or affection. Treatment may be most helpful when it allows the incest survivor to regain a sense of control through insight and support. Another important assumption is that a clinician has a responsibility to develop some awareness about his/her internal reactions to incest, and therefore, not send any messages that interfere with resolution (for example, that incest is a secret to be kept or a behavior to be condemned).

Adults molested as children (AMAC) groups have been identified as a popular and useful part of treatment (Gagliano, 1987; Gordy, 1983). These groups have been used along with individual psychotherapy groups for the purpose of this study. The author has found that groups allow survivors to be taken seriously, to feel less isolated, to learn about typical reactions, and to practice new skills.

Stages of Incest Trauma Resolution

The six stages identified as part of incest trauma resolution are denial, shame, fight or flight, depression, acceptance, and repairing damage. Descriptions of the stages are discussed in the following paragraphs. A list of the stages can be presented to the client and/or group for discussion, to serve as the base for a common language and focus for treatment.

Stage 1: Denial

The first stage is denial. When survivors deny their incest experience or its impact, they are displaying incorporation of societal attitudes (Forward & Buck, 1978) and activation of defense mechanisms to protect against unresolved conflict or unacceptable feelings (Freud, 1946). When survivors enter treatment, they commonly say, "I can't remember much of my childhood." However, there often is actual repression of memories along with occasional nightmares, hallucinations, or flashbacks representing disassociated pieces of those memories (Ellenson, 1985).

Society's incest taboo can be a powerful factor reinforcing denial. Although the incest taboo is adaptive for survival purposes (Forward

& Buck, 1978), it fosters denial because no one wants to be the object of social judgment or disgust. Some mental health professionals may reinforce denial because of their socialized attitudes of horror toward incest and discomfort with human sexuality. They may be slow to acknowledge the reality of incest, tend to miss its signals, and also to downplay its significance in the diagnostic picture (Courtois & Watts, 1982; Forward & Buck, 1978).

Denial may be used intrapsychically as a defense mechanism to protect against overwhelming, unacceptable, or painful feelings. One client never thought about her sexual abuse and just pretended that it never happened, until she got so depressed that she required hospitalization. When confronted with actual memories, clients may say "Why dig up the past? I want to go on from here and forget the bad things." This is similar to the reaction of dying patients discussed by Kübler-Ross (1969) in her stages-of-grief work, where denial is seen as a healthy way to deal with an unchanging, painful situation.

Many clients move out of denial when they experience therapy as a safe place where they have permission to have and share their "secret." This is done by taking the client and what she/he presents seriously, asking matter-of-fact questions, and naming the experience for what it is.

Once denial is overcome, clients often **Stage 2: Shame** begin to experience considerable shame and guilt. They anticipate severe judgment and condemnation from others. They talk of "feeling dirty" and responsible, saying "I shouldn't have let it happen." They remember having always felt different from peers, especially in school, and frightened that others might discover the terrible secret about them. This secret may not be the incest experience itself, but something related to their coping mechanisms (for example, suicide attempts, hallucinations, eating disorders, or substance abuse). They may remember certain scenes and play back repeatedly what they "should have done" instead of "letting it happen." They often feel that they have betrayed the perpetrator or the family by disclosing the secret and feel deserving of punishment. The goal here, as noted by Forward and Buck (1978) in their discussion of treatment issues, is to "help the victim place the responsibility for the incest firmly where it belongs . . . with the adult . . ." (p. 167). As noted by Gagliano (1987), the victim has often been told by an aggressor that she/he "is bad, seductive, or responsible for the adult's sexual behavior" (p. 102). Group treatment has been recognized as a powerful medium for helping to reduce shame and guilt (Gagliano, 1987). The source of the guilt may have to do with the pleasure gained by attention, privilege, affection, or physical contact. Members can see that their peers are not responsible for the abuse and can translate this to themselves.

Once responsibility for the act of incest is squarely placed on the shoulders of the aggressor, survivors seem to get in touch with

**Stage 3:
Fight or Flight**

feelings of rage at the perpetrator and significant others who did not protect them from abuse. The rage can become intense and frightening, leading survivors toward decompensation or a move back to stage one of denial in order to contain these feelings. Treatment at this point requires careful monitoring for evidence of self-destructive behavior and active structuring of outlets for anger.

Survivors in a group at this point may tend to transfer their anger to the group therapist, representative of the authority figure who did not protect or hear their needs. The therapist can recognize and clarify the feelings directed at him or her by the client for "not saying/reaching out enough" (being absent) or "intruding/dominating too much" (being abusive). Interpreting the connections to the primary experience can lead to increased insight. Kübler-Ross (1969) noted this displacement process during the stage of anger. She suggests that grievances against helping personnel should not be taken personally and require patience and understanding.

When some of the anger is spent, survivors often move into sadness and depression. They start to get in touch with their

**Stage 4:
Depression**

losses, especially the loss of innocence, the sense of never having a childhood, and the loss of trust that anyone was available to protect or care for them in the environment. Basic trust can be damaged badly. Survivors experience feeling lost, alone, and empty—a deep sense of isolation that has followed them for many years. Sharing this in a group can help to vent the pain of feeling alone and provide a connection to others. It is important at this stage to validate the losses and the pain instead of trying to make it go away (Kübler-Ross, 1969).

When survivors hear about the acceptance stage in the beginning of treatment, they often wonder if it will ever come. Ac-

**Stage 5:
Acceptance**

ceptance is present when there is a feeling of greater internal strength and self-awareness. There is less of a focus on the status of "victim."

As Kübler-Ross (1969) discusses the acceptance stage of dying, there is a sense of inner peace as the struggle and pain diminish. Survivors will no longer punish themselves by dwelling in or holding onto the pain of their experience.

Acceptance, along with the other stages, does not invariably appear in perfect timing and order. Survivors report experiencing aspects of more than one stage at a time. However, there is usually a primary focus of the emotional intensity at any given time. When survivors arrive at the acceptance stage, they are not immune from reexperiencing affect related to previous stages, especially when prompted by appropriate environmental stimuli.

Stage 6: Repairing Damage

Even when normal feelings about the incest experience have been worked through, survivors often make statements such as "but there's more to deal with; people always seem to take advantage of or hurt me; I feel helpless to get my needs heard or met in relationships; I'm scared of being close; I can't say no or assert myself." This type of response may be evidence of ongoing damage that must be repaired for final resolution of the incest impact. Incest teaches certain types of survival skills during the time of childhood when other skills should have been learned. Incest victims learn how to take care of others in order to get their needs met, how to suppress their assertiveness, how to use sex to obtain attention or affection, and how to develop control of their mind and feelings because they are powerless to control their physical safety or boundaries. These survival skills are dysfunctional when they reach adulthood. They may need to learn self-defense skills, assertiveness skills, how to experience pleasure without guilt or self-punishment, and awareness of their emotional needs as deserving of gratification.

A program of skill building around these issues is recommended to increase a client's functioning level, even if the client is unable to tolerate a focus on stages 1 through 5 because of a disrupted or disorganized sense of self. With vulnerable psychiatric populations, this phase of skill building may be helpful to develop a foundation for further work or when other types of work are not possible. Thus, social workers can use the six stages to help clients move from being self-destructive victims to being productive survivors.

Case Examples

Case of B

B is a 22-year-old single female who was referred to a community mental health center by a rape hotline when she began to have nightmares and flashes of memory about incest with her mother. She became frightened and depressed and was unable to concentrate on school or work and cried frequently. She recently had begun a new lesbian relationship where she was afraid of being dominated. She remained in treatment for about one year with a combination of individual and group therapy. *Denial Stage:* When she entered treatment, B had maintained denial by forgetting and repressing memories of severe sexual abuse that continued from age 5 to 13. She recovered memories piece by piece throughout the first nine months of treatment. She reported that being taken seriously about her experience was the most valuable aspect of treatment because it allowed her to face memories and stop denying what had happened. *Shame Stage:* The shame and guilt she felt centered around being passive instead of somehow stopping the abuse. This feeling was present even though she acknowledged being physically overpowered. She remembered that as a child she had the ever-present idea that she was a bad girl and deserved punishment. She punished herself with stoicism—seeing how many pleasurable things she could withhold from herself to gain a sense of control and pride (for example, not eating ice cream because it tasted good to her). *Fight or Flight Stage:* Her rage during treatment exploded in some "tantrums" at home where she screamed and cried hysterically for about an hour at a time. In sessions, she voiced intense anger at her mother: "How dare she hurt and abuse me?" "Why won't she admit it now when confronted?" and "How dare she cheat me out of being a normal kid!" *Depression Stage:* B cried extensively with pain and sadness about a childhood where she often felt scared, bad, and unloved. *Acceptance Stage:* Finally, she was able to say to herself, "Yes, it really happened, it wasn't my fault, and I deserve better." *Repairing Damage Stage:* B anguished about her difficulty with feeling a part of groups and her tendency to allow people to walk over her by giving them whatever they asked for. "You mean I can say no without being attacked?" she asked. The last phase of her treatment focused on communication and assertiveness issues with her partner and friends where she learned to rebuild trust and assert her needs.

S is a 34-year-old divorced female, in- **Case of S**
voluntarily hospitalized because of severe
depression, suicidal impulses, and a recent fire in her home. During the fire, she had awakened at home with her two children to the smell of smoke and was worried she may have set the fire without remembering it. She suffered from severe depression, which included episodes of active suicide attempts, self-mutilation, periods of

amnesia, and violent hallucinations filled with blood and terror. She was seen in an inpatient psychiatric unit for four months. *Denial Stage:* She pretended that the severe physical abuse by her mother and sexual abuse by her father from age 13 to 16 never happened and put it out of her mind. *Shame Stage:* In treatment, she reported her history in a matter-of-fact way. She first experienced relief and support but then became frightened and withdrawn, filled with fear of rejection by those who would know her secret. In her AMAC group, she was appalled that a fellow member let slip an identification to peers on the unit about the content of the group. Her guilt centered on her suicide attempts (not being strong enough to cope), episodes of cutting on herself with razors (being so "stupid"), and inability to care well for her children, leading to possible loss of custody. *Fight or Flight Stage:* In group, she shared with peers about her experience and asked "Why would a mother tell her own daughter she is ugly?" This focus first on rage over a lack of maternal protection or support is common. A few days later, as she heard stories of sexual abuse by peers, she began to experience rage in the form of a fantasy of murdering her father, methodically planning and executing it down to the last detail. This fantasy felt real and she became terrified of losing control. *Depression Stage:* She became severely depressed and experienced violent hallucinations, extreme self-contempt, head banging, urges to self-multilate, and slowed psychomotor functioning. She was informed that staff would not allow her to hurt herself. The forms of protection including medication, suicide watch, restricted community passes, and possible transfer to a more secure facility were discussed. All of these were used except for transfer out. She was able to maintain sufficient control and voiced a desire not to be transferred because she had become attached and did not want to lose the help she felt was available in the form of therapy and peer support. *Acceptance Stage:* She gradually recovered from the depression, emerging with a sense of increased strength, and moved on to a transitional living program where she planned to attend a day treatment program. *Repairing Damage:* Evidence of damage to trust and interactional skills was pervasive and would require long-term outpatient care.

Case of T

T is a 30-year-old single female involuntarily hospitalized for depression with a suicide attempt. She revealed that she had been molested at age 13 by a friend of her father. She was subsequently raped by a stranger (one year before her hospitalization) and recently had begun to experience nightmares (flashbacks of the scenes of rape and molestation at night while sleeping, which led to sudden awakening with severe anxiety).

She was treated in an inpatient psychiatric unit for two months with medication, group, individual, and an AMAC group that focused only on repairing damage. She attended a total of five group sessions dealing with themes of safety, trust, assertiveness, and self-care. The treatment focus was on setting goals and building skills about current difficulties in the various areas of damage or deficit stemming from incest or sexual assault experiences. *Repairing Damage:* T identified goals about reducing the frequency of her nightmares and telling people directly when they say things that hurt her. In discussing her nightmares, the focus was on how she could feel safer both by day and night. She was able to identify at what times she felt safe and how she created a sense of safety (for example, by going out in public only when accompanied by someone instead of alone). Her attempts to increase safety were recognized and reinforced. Brainstorming with the group led to a list of ways people can increase their safety. Attention to her nightmares focused on how best to take care of herself around them, or how to elicit comfort or reassurance for herself. T reported that her nightmares had decreased by the end of her stay. In helping her to tell people her reactions directly, the group role played and provided feedback to help her practice communicating in effective ways. She was teased by a group member who called her a "conehead." T was able to say she felt hurt and ask the peer not to say things like that because she was sensitive.

Comparison of Inpatient and Outpatient

There are certain similarities between inpatient and outpatient AMAC groups. The members of both appear to bond quickly and develop a strong sense of cohesion based on their common experience. The emotional and motivational levels are usually high, leading to intense and productive work as the norm. Both types of groups require careful preparation of members. This is especially true in an inpatient unit, where rules such as confidentiality take on greater significance. In addition, both groups require readiness for entry. Identifying where a client is functioning in terms of the stages of incest resolution can facilitate the use of appropriate timing for group entry. Clients who are solidly out of denial and struggling with shame may be the best candidates for a group. A client with an overwhelmingly chaotic lifestyle, an active substance abuse problem, a life-threatening eating disorder, or a current life crisis may not be ready for group treatment on incest impact.

There are some essential differences in an inpatient AMAC group. First of all, the length of stay is short (often 60 days or less) and there is rapid turnover of group members. The group members will have contact with many different staff who have varying levels of sensitivity to their needs. Training and consultation with staff by the group leader is advised.

In addition, there is generally a lower level of ego strengths and functioning. Some survivors were never able to attend any groups due to the severity of symptoms they experienced because reality contact was too limited to provide more than basic custodial care. Certain schizophrenic and bipolar disordered clients were able to attend a group. They seemed to benefit from a feeling of belonging as part of an identified group. They valued the support and were able to participate in skill-building exercises even if discussion comments were loose or difficult to follow. Exercises and discussions were geared to their level of functioning and varied depending on group members present at any given session.

A structured, time-limited group for the inpatient treatment setting was designed, with different topic areas to be covered each week. The topics included: safety, assertiveness, building trust, and taking care of yourself. Group members set goals related to these topics and worked on building the skills they needed, with structure and support supplied by the group leader. There was an intention to focus away from stages 1 through 5, putting primary clinical investment into building up ego strengths and skills. Further resolution of the stages may be done in outpatient or longer term work.

Implications for Treatment and Research

There remain many questions about treatment for incest survivors. For example, when a client has multiple problems, how does one decide the relative impact or importance of the incest issues? Does the theory of stages presented here really serve a predictive function for all or some segment of incest survivors? The stages have appeared to be helpful in organizing clinical perceptions and treatment interventions, but may be best used as one part of an overall treatment approach based on psychosocial needs and personality factors.

Treatment of incest is not a simple task. It can be complicated by layers of other intrapsychic and environmental problems. It also can be sabotaged in the public sector when agencies short of staff and funding are reluctant to use precious treatment resources for one special population when there are so many competing priorities and special needs with which they must contend. Conceding to these limitations, it is commendable that many mental health professionals see the need and respond to incest cases competently with various treatment techniques. It is hoped that the assessment/treatment approach presented in this article may be a useful addition and a basis for further work in the field.

References

Benward, J., & Densen-Gerber, J. (1975). Incest as a causative factor in antisocial behavior: An exploratory study. *Contemporary Drug Problems, 4,* 323–340.

Courtois, C. A., & Watts, D. L. (1982). Counseling adult women who experienced incest in childhood and adolescence. *Personnel and Guidance Journal, 60,* 275–279.

Ellenson, G. S. (1985). Detecting a history of incest: A predictive syndrome. *Social Casework: The Journal of Contemporary Social Work, 66,* 525–532.

Ellenson, G. S. (1986). Disturbances of perception in adult female incest survivors. *Social Casework: The Journal of Contemporary Social Work, 67,* 149–159.

Erikson, E. H. (1963). *Childhood and society.* New York: W. W. Norton.

Forward, S., & Buck, C. (1978). *Betrayal of innocence.* New York: Penguin Books.

Freud, A. (1946). *The ego and mechanisms of defense.* New York: International Universities Press.

Gagliano, C. K. (1987). Group treatment for sexually abused girls. *Social Casework: The Journal of Contemporary Social Work, 2,* 102–108.

Gelinas, D. J. (1983). Persisting negative effects of incest. *Psychiatry, 46,* 312–332.

Gordy, P. L. (1983). Group work that supports adult victims of childhood incest. *Social Casework: The Journal of Contemporary Social Work, 64,* 300–307.

Kübler-Ross, E. (1969). *On death and dying.* New York: MacMillan.

Rosenfeld, A. A. (1979). Incidence of history of incest among 18 female psychiatric patients. *American Journal of Psychiatry, 136,* 791–795.

Vander Mey, B. J., & Neff, R. L. (1982). Adult–child incest—A review of research and treatment. *Adolescence, 17,* 715–733.

CHRONIC ILLNESS AND THE QUALITY OF LIFE:
The Social Worker's Role

Shirley A. Conger and Kay D. Moore

T he extraordinary extension of life in the twentieth century
brings in its wake new problems—namely, an increase in
chronic illness and the need for long-term care. Accelerating
advances in medical and biological technology and practice
have brought concomitant problems associated with longevity. The major factor in the prevalence of long-term illness is the impressive elimination or control of infectious and parasitic diseases.
These have been replaced by the degenerative diseases of the aging
population. The result of these technological advances is that chronic
illness has become the major challenge to all health professionals. The
aim of health improvement must be the management of chronic illness
with the goal of enhancing not only the length but the quality of life
(McGlone, 1982).

The Commission on Chronic
Illness in 1956 provided the
following definition of *chronic
disease:*

Chronic Illness and the Quality of Life in Old Age

All impairments or deviations from normal which have one or more of the following characteristics: are permanent, leave residual disability, are caused by non-reversible pathological alteration, require special training of the patient for rehabilitation, may be expected to require a long period of supervision, observation or care. (Mayo, 1956, p. 9)

Although only 14 percent of those over 65 are free of chronic illness, the great majority of the elderly live independently in their own homes. It is the old, those over 80 years, who have increasing frailty and multiple chronic illnesses, who are the at-risk group. The health, social, and economic problems of the elderly, especially those over age 75, are predominantly problems concerning women. Life expectancy of men is less than that for women and men are more likely to have family supports. Old age is associated with women living alone on reduced income and in increased poverty, accompanied with a greater risk of ill health, institutionalization, and death (Lamy, 1986a).

Social policy regarding long-term care of the frail elderly in the United States has exhibited a perceptible bias toward institutional care and away from community care since the passage of the Medicare and Medicaid provisions of the Social Security Act (Scharlach & Frenzel, 1986). In the future, the care of the chronically ill must shift toward alternatives to institutionalization.

Some of the major and complicated problems of living with chronic illness include the management of crises, handling of regimens, controlling of symptoms, mitigating of social isolation, and aiding of the attempt to live normally and maintain normal social relations. Coupled with these challenges are the normal losses of aging: vision, hearing, and other sensory deficits; reduction in energy; narrowing of social opportunities; and gradually increasing dependence on others.

Specific chronic conditions and their implications include the crippling conditions and pain of rheumatoid arthritis and osteoarthritis, progressive renal failure, emphysema, incontinence, congestive heart failure, stroke, cancer (which has become a chronic disease), and gastrointestinal disorders. Many elderly individuals are hospitalized not for acute disease but because they are experiencing an acute phase of a chronic condition. Moreover, frequently the person suffers from multiple chronic diseases in which the treatment for one may have negative side effects for another (Viney & Westbrook, 1981). These conditions require a delicate balancing of medical, social, and psychological adjustments to the changing reality of current health status.

Although the detailed medical discussions of etiology, symptomatology, treatment, and regimens often have social consequences for the elderly person and the family, generally there is not much focus on how that person and the family might better manage their lives, given the particular disease and long-term care needs. There is little focus, either, on how social workers might help with the problems that come in the wake of chronic illness and its treatments—problems such as social stigmatization of the ill person, isolation, family disruption, marital discord, transformation of domestic roles, or how to prevent fatal physiological crises through making necessary arrangements with the family or other caregivers.

One of the unmentionables about the elderly is their decreased sexual function and corresponding decrease in the quality of life. Sexuality is adversely affected by both chronic illnesses and drug side effects. The unspoken assumption that elderly people are asexual prevents the recognition of the problem and its solution.

Psychological Reactions to Chronic Illness

Patients who suffer disability as a result of chronic illness react psychologically in a variety of ways. The pattern of reaction has been reported to contain the following nine elements (Viney & Westbrook, 1981):

1. Uncertainty.
2. Anxiety.
3. Depression.
4. Anger expressed directly.
5. Anger expressed indirectly. The effective disruption and tension have been found to occur regardless of the severity of the illness.
6. Competence—a feeling for which all patients strive even when their illness is life threatening.
7. Helplessness and hopelessness, emotions that few patients can avoid.
8. Threatened sociability.
9. Good feelings may vary as a function of the patient's disability.

It is difficult to predict a patient's reaction to disability, but in general the more global the disabling condition, the more devastating it is psychologically. Persons who are particularly vulnerable are persons with limited education and, conversely, those with high occupational status. Chronic illness will trigger much uncertainty and related depression (McGlone, 1982). Chronic illness is related to anomie, a feeling of powerlessness and social isolation. The following items are considered characteristic of anomie: (1) indifference of community leaders; (2) unpredictability of the social order; (3) impossibility of the realization of life goals; (4) sense of the meaninglessness of life; and (5) immediate personal relationships are no longer predictive or supportive (cannot count even on one's closest friends) (Ben-Sira, 1984).

The stress–illness relationship serves **Stress and** to highlight the health-deteriorating effect **Coping** of chronic illness. Illness constitutes an expression of "breakdown" due to a prolonged failure of restoring a person's emotional homeostasis. The impact of chronic illness on a person's emotional homeostasis is predominantly at the perceptual level—to a great extent it is not the demand per se, but rather the individual's assessment of it that makes the demand a stressor. The same experience may be highly threatening to one person, yet harmless to another. According to this approach, any illness, acute or chronic, is conceived as an expression of breakdown (Ben-Sira, 1984).

For the chronically ill, self-controlled resources are more effective than other-controlled resources. This conforms with theories of stress and breakdown: whatever the demands, ultimately it is the individual who is constantly confronted by them, interprets them, assigns them a subjective meaning, and constantly has to respond to them. The greater an individual's control of resources, the greater will be his or her capacity to cope successfully.

Dependence on the environment for meeting the demands has at least two disadvantages that make them less effective than self-controlled resources. First, because their proximity is not omnipresent, chances are that one may be confronted with demands in the absence of the appropriate "environmental resources," and thus be unable to meet them at the time of their occurrence. Second, getting help, and hence "buying" resources from the social environment, incurs a "cost" on the "buyer," such as admission of his or her inferior status, or giving certain services in return for the help given. This reduces the "net profit" of the exchange.

There will be, however, demands requiring other-controlled resources. In this respect, primary group support has an advantage over that of the secondary social environment, in particular over professional support, by being based on a reciprocal affective relationship. The mere membership of a person in a primary group, by definition, implies a person's value for that group and has the stress-buffering role of social support by a person's primary social network such as family and friends. Help proferred by a professional results in a sense of inferiority and powerlessness vis-a-vis a "powerful professional," a sense that is inherent in the dependence on the needed assistance, on the one hand, and on the professional's striving to maintain and enhance his or her power on the other (Ben-Sira, 1984).

The indispensibility of professional help highlights his or her dependence on that help for responding to a vital demand, thus implying inferiority. The chronically ill person has to cope with new demands that may arise from permanent incapacitation, which is frequently accompanied by stigma and the constant fear of a possible occurrence of additional episodes with further damaging results, and with the potential of depriving that person abruptly or gradually of control over his or her entire life. The afflicted individual and his or her primary network may feel helpless and incompetent to affect his or her physical condition substantially. They may be explicitly aware of their incompetence of coping also with the emotional disturbance that may result from physical and medical problems.

Any effort at improving or at least arresting deterioration of the physical and emotional state may point to the need for help of professionals such as social workers. This dependence and sense of powerlessness is deleterious to one's well-being and contradictory to the restoration of emotional homeostasis. Given these parameters, the social worker must strive to increase the subject's area of control and to maintain the right to decision making.

Patients judge the quality of the treatment and the physician's competence, and gain reassurance from the physician's affective behavior toward them. However, in light of the dominance of the biomedical model in medical practice, the physician focuses on physical disturbance rather than on the emotional state of the afflicted individual. Doctors can be hindered profoundly by some aspects of their professional training in understanding and paying attention to the patient's emotional problems. The physician tends to view the patient's anxiety as an outcome of the disease, which will "naturally" be alleviated upon recovery from the illness. Indeed, emotional support is not seen by doctors as professionally challenging.

Moreover, the physician's recognition of an inability to help (that is, cure) the patient medically may constitute a sense of failure. That in turn may lead to defensive behavior by avoiding as much as possible confronting the patient, a behavior that frequently is justified by the necessity to allocate the scarce resources (the doctor's time) mainly to those who are likely to benefit the most from the doctor's intervention. The patient may interpret the physician's avoidance of him or her as indifference, and consequently may feel deserted. The chronically ill person appears to be highly vulnerable to further deterioration of his or her or her condition, not merely because of progressive damage caused by the illness itself, but because of the emotional disturbance owing to the inefficacy of the person's individual and primary group resources and the perceived indifference of the physician. The social worker's task can be that of clarifying these feelings so they can be dealt with by the patient, family, and physician.

Since the seventeenth century, a first **Disease–Illness** principle of medical practice has been the **Paradigm** mandate to define the one disease that underlies a patient's distress. Treatment directed at this underlying disease represents the most direct and effective way to alleviate symptoms. Despite the overwhelming success of this disease–illness paradigm, its limitations cannot be disregarded: many diseases do not necessarily produce illness, and the quality of the illness may not be predictable from knowledge of the disease. For example, knowing the extent of disease in a patient with rheumatoid arthritis does not allow one to predict confidently the capacity of that patient to work. The search for reversible disease, although important, is a secondary issue in the management of chronic illness and may even be detrimental to helping the patient live more comfortably (Williams & Hadler, 1983).

Often, iatrogenous problems (especially drug toxicities and abuse of physical restraints) are the reversible processes identified. A disease-specific focus deemphasizes the dominant issue in the management of chronic illness, which is the maximization of the patient's productivity, creativity, well-being, and happiness. This goal of improving patient function and satisfaction to the fullest extent is usually achieved without curing the underlying disease. In chronic illness of the elderly, information meaningful in the definition of disease is elusive.

The third argument for defining disease in the chronically ill is to allow accurate prognosis, which is useful in estimating longevity. Small reductions in life expectancy become nearly irrelevant in the elderly. Even for some less-chronic problems, many patients seem to prefer improved quality of life over extended life span.

Most of the disability experienced by the elderly results from diseases that represent exaggerations of normal age-related physiologic decline. Three examples illustrate the assertion that the definition of the underlying disease often is not critical in the management or assessment of most chronic illness in the elderly (Williams & Hadler, 1983). These are as follows:

1. Urinary incontinence is the involuntary loss of quantities of urine sufficient to be a social or hygienic problem. It may be due to sphincter weakness or some other bladder condition, to reduced mobility, or to iatrogenous sources such as restraints or medications.

2. Approximately three-fourths of elderly patients suffer lower-back pain. Particularly in the elderly backaches compromise the ability to care for oneself (inability to dress and maintain personal control to move about, and to retrieve objects); the results can be confinement as well as the loss of independence in functioning. Despite the prevalence of lower-back pain, physicians only rarely identify a specific underlying cause. Consequently, lower-back pain is an example

of an illness in search of a disease. The management of lower-back pain involves educating the patient and recommending adjustment of the environment, exercise, and low doses of aspirin or other nonsteroidal and anti-inflammatory agents. The definition of underlying disease is rarely accomplished, and, if it is, it is rarely rewarding. Even more humbling is the fact that many features of backache depend more on psychosocial influences than on disease elements.

3. Manual dexterity, in one highly selected subset of elderly women, appears to be intimately and principally associated with the ability to live independently. The quantification of manual inefficiency in elderly patients provides important information for making clinical decisions that relate to the probability that the patient will lose independence.

Understanding the difference between illness and disease is a prerequisite to the care of patients affected by incurable disorders. Even though many chronic conditions are incurable, the discomfort or disability they produce may be substantially modified.

Family Illness Rituals

Rituals are repeated patterns of behavior that often contain deeply compacted meanings. Families have rituals for dealing with many aspects of life and among these are rituals for dealing with illness. Just as an individual's daily habits reflect his or her inner conflicts, so a family's rituals can condense and express its beliefs, images, style, and role assignments. Further, they provide models for dealing with sickness that are passed down from generation to generation. Sensitivity to such patterns can attune the social worker to basic family dynamics (Glenn, 1982).

At the heart of family illness rituals is the issue of caretaking. Who takes care of the sick or of the caretaker? Do both members of a couple care for one another in times of illness, or is the relationship fixed in one direction only? What happens to a family when a previously healthy member falls ill? How long does the family take to recognize an illness? Who recognizes it? What does it take to qualify as sick and what must happen to warrant going to a physician? What weight does the physician's pronouncement carry in the family? Often, the way a couple first handles illness in one of its members sets a pattern that may endure for years (Glenn, 1982).

Families that must cope with chronic illnesses can be transformed by the task. They start accepting the accoutrements of illness as family objects and develop rituals of handling them. Such is the case of an invalid's wheelchair, for instance. Where is it kept? Whose job is it to care for it? Does the same family member always wheel the invalid about, or do several take turns? Does the invalid insist on being "independent," or is the illness an occasion for greater claim for assistance? How does the wheelchair restrict where the patient can go—to people's homes, to the bathroom, to the physician's office?

Rituals connected with severe illness include such things as visits to the hospital, patterned family interaction with the physician, and, in cases where death attends, the "vigil." A crisis encountered in an acute illness usually requires the family to reorganize itself, to bury minor discontents for a time, and to present a unified front. Many families know who should take charge during an episode of illness. Some families restructure themselves in the face of illness; still others may be unable to come together as a result of old conflicts that may actually deepen.

Determining these kinds of family interactions is the area of expertise of the social worker whose job it is to interpret them to other members of the health-care team.

The Elderly and Drug Interactions

Information on drug interactions in the elderly and their possible clinical sequelae is still incomplete. Adverse drug reactions occur more often and are more severe in the elderly because of altered drug distribution (loss of weight, change in lean body weight/lipid tissue), metabolism (altered liver function), and excretion (changed renal function), the latter factor being most important. An altered homeostatic mechanism accounts for an elderly patient's lessened ability to compensate for adverse drug effects. Most are predictable and, therefore, avoidable, by adjustment of dose or administration times, or by selection of an appropriate alternate drug. The drugs most often involved are not necessarily new and exotic drugs, but old and well-known chronic-care drugs such as diuretics, warfarin, digoxin, oral hypoglycemics, H2-histamine blockers, and nonsteroidals. Not all drug interactions result in adverse effects, and some can be beneficial if properly managed (Lamy, 1982b, 1986; Sloan, 1983).

The potential for drug interactions increases tremendously with the number of medications prescribed. When two drugs are used in combination, the possibility of an interaction is 5.6 percent; for five drugs, the rate is 50 percent. When eight drugs are prescribed together, the potential for an interaction is 100 percent (Table 1) (Lamy, 1986).

Those age 65 and older face almost twice the chance of iatrogenic disease than do younger patients, and they usually visit physician offices more often than young people, mostly because of chronic

Table 1
**Effects of Multiple-Drug Use on the Incidence
of Adverse Reactions**

	Number of Drugs Prescribed			
	0–5	6–10	11–15	16–20
Patients	4,009	3,861	1,713	641
Adverse reactions				
Total	142	397	478	347
Percent	4	10	28	54

SOURCE: May, Stewart, and Leighton, 1977.

diseases. Seventy percent of those age 75 and older receive drugs. Of the 25 most-often used drugs, 11 are antihypertensive or cardiac drugs. The use of nonsteroidals increases sharply with advancing age.

Lack of supervision of long-term care drugs used in management of chronic diseases is one of the major reasons for problems the elderly have with their drugs. Yet supervision is needed to a much larger degree than given, because the frequency of drug interactions rises and falls with the number of drugs prescribed. In a group of geriatric patients, the rate of adverse drug reactions (and, presumably, interactions) fell from 24.3 percent to 7 percent when the average number of drugs per patient was decreased from 7.8 to 6.9 (Sloan, 1983). The orally administered anticoagulants probably have the greatest potential of any pharmacologic class of drugs for clinically significant interactions with other drugs.

Of major importance for the elderly wishing to retain an independent status is mental acuity. Many drugs are common causes of transient cognitive disorders such as delirium and acute confusional states, as well as anxiety, depression, insomnia, or undue sedation. Included in the list of drugs are such frequently used drugs for the elderly as diuretics, analgesics, antihistamines, antiparkinsonian agents, antidepressents, beta blockers, and other cardiovascular drugs, neuroleptics, cimetidine, and digitalis (Cupit, 1982; Greenblatt, Divoll, Abernethy, & Shader, 1982).

Nonprescription Drugs and Drug Interactions

A large percentage of over-the-counter drugs are purchased by the elderly. It has been reported that only 37 percent of patients ever ask the pharmacist for advice before purchasing a nonprescription product. Many patients do not read the nonprescription drug warning labels, and even if they did, many of the instructions are written at a level incomprehensible to the general public. People do not consider nonprescription products "drugs." When the family physician asks patients what drugs they are taking, it is only the rare patient who will remember, or even consider it important enough, to mention such nonprescription medications as pain relievers, vitamins, laxatives, cough/cold preparations, or diet aids. For example, the salicylates (aspirin and other similar medications) can lead to toxic reactions such as confusion, irritability, vision disturbances, sweating, nausea, vomiting, diarrhea, and lowering of temperature. Combined use of aspirin and other drugs may lead to accidental hypothermia (Rose, 1985; Lamy, 1982a).

Drug Risks

Realization of drug risks mandates a closer monitoring function to be shared by the physician, pharmacist, nurses, social workers, and the patient. Is the patient able to communicate? Is he or she able to use a telephone or hear instructions? A current assessment of mental status is important here (Lamy, 1982a).

Dementia

About 5 percent of Americans over age 65 (more than one million) are afflicted by dementia to the extent that they are unable to care for themselves. Another 10 percent suffer from milder degrees of this disorder. There may, in fact, be as many as 50 different causes of dementia, and perhaps 20 percent of all dementias are secondary to treatable causes. Thus, management of the elderly with dementia requires that there be an accurate diagnosis and treatment (if possible) and a realistic prognosis (Gershon & Herman, 1982). The two principal causes of irreversible dementia are Alzheimer's disease and multiple infarction. With accurate diagnosis, the family can make a realistic plan for care.

Pseudodementia and Depression

The incidence of depression is probably the most common of all the psychiatric syndromes. Its prevalence rates in the elderly may range from 10 to 50 percent depending on the population surveyed. The risk of depression increases with age, with women at higher risk than men until after age 65, when the risks are equal. There also is a close connection between physical illness and depression in the geriatric population: 30 to 50 percent of the elderly who have physical diseases also have affective disorders. In addition, although people over age 65 constitute about 11 percent of the population, they account for 25 percent of all suicides. In depression, thought processes are often slow and the content morbid and guilt ridden. The affect is sad and despairing. Disturbances of appetite, sleep, weight, and energy may occur. The person may become agitated or retarded in motor behavior (Gershon & Herman, 1982).

Depression may be masked by somatic complaints such as fatigue, sexual dysfunction, or chronic pain. The presenting complaint may be impairment of memory or thought processes. Certain general features help distinguish pseudodementia from true dementia. Pseudodementia is accompanied generally by changes in sleep, appetite, and energy level. There is often a history of affective illness. Patients with pseudodementia tend to emphasize their disabilities, are able to provide detailed histories of their cognitive deficits, and are usually upset by them. Those patients with true dementias, such as Alzheimer's disease, often attempt to conceal their disabilities or act unconcerned. Patients with pseudodementia respond to treatment, whereas those with true dementias do not (Grieco & Kopel, 1983).

Self-Help and Self-Care in Chronic Illness

Today, nonprofessionals directly provide about 75 percent of the health care needed for themselves and their families, without professional intervention. The rising interest in self-help coincides with a shift in medical treatment goals from cure to management and maintenance of an acceptable quality of life. The emphasis in patient care has changed to management of permanent, chronic, or terminal conditions such as heart disease and cancer (Strauss & Glaser, 1975).

The chief business of the chronically ill person is not just to stay alive or keep symptoms under control, but to live as normally as possible. How normal that life (and that of the family) can be depends not only on the social arrangements that can be made but on how intrusive are the symptoms, medical regimens, and knowledge others have of the person's disease. Care must be taken by members of the team to help the patient avoid changes that can threaten the delicate fabric of normality that has been created. Especially difficult is the task of maintaining normal relationships when people know that the disease is fatal. This knowledge and the fear it strikes in others can be a major obstacle to open, normal communication. A "closed awareness" or secrecy often becomes the policy of family members who are experiencing the anguish of anticipatory grief over the potential loss. Persons who have visible manifestations of illness or stigmata of illness have an especially difficult challenge to maintaining normal relationships.

A significant problem for all chronically ill persons is the necessary reordering of time (Schilling & Schilling, 1987). Even a simple

operation such as a trip to the doctor, store, or a social event may require careful planning to conserve energy, arrive on time to get a seat,
arrange for transportation, and present a normal, self-contained appearance. This management of time and of normal functioning requires enormous amounts of self-control, planning, and supports that
are not obtrusive. The management of medical regimens also poses
difficulties. Failure to do so is often regarded by health-care personnel as deliberate noncompliance or lack of cooperation, with the result
of disapproval of the patient and family. However, the issue is not just
stupidity or unwillingness, but that the combined load is too much for
the coping ability of the sick person.

Regimens are not accepted automatically and are adhered to only if there is continuing trust in the doctor who prescribes the regimen;
no rival supersedes the doctor; there is evidence that the regimen
works either to control symptoms or the disease or both; no distress-
ing, frightening side affects appear, such as severe pain, excessive
nausea, dizziness, or lethargy; the side effects or risks are outweighed
by symptom relief or by sufficient fear of the disease itself; there is
little interference with important daily activities either of the sick person or those around him or her; and the perceived good effects are not
outweighed by a negative impact on the person's sense of identity
(Strauss & Glaser, 1975).

Learning how to work with new machines or implements can be
anxiety provoking, and therefore, all health-care personnel need to
give the sick person enough support to allow them and the caregiver
to master these techniques with confidence.

Social Worker as a Member of the Health-Care Team

Given the complexities of
chronic illness and aging itself, the
social worker cannot be effective
working alone, but must function
as a member of a health-care team, in which the social worker acts
as a patient advocate and as an educator about psychosocial needs.
Also, because the chronically ill elderly person needs medical,
psychological, and social support, the challenge is to provide this
without being perceived as patronizing or in any way demeaning to
the already fragile ego of the vulnerable client/patient. Social workers
are beginning to recognize that as their interventions can be helpful,
so can they be harmful. Concern for the client cannot, in itself, justify
social intervention. Potential benefits must outweigh likely risks. As
social workers are better able to identify such risks, they may have
more influence over patient care (Schilling & Schilling, 1987). It may
be that the rule "less is more" applies; the goal is always the least

restrictive environment. In many cases, the social worker may be more effective as a case manager or a counselor to the care providers, helping them procure needed services such as special equipment and respite care for themselves.

Other areas of expertise are client and family support groups, therapy groups, discharge planning, community outreach, and volunteer programs. The social worker must be aware always of the changing level of functioning of the ill elderly client—last month's assessment may be entirely unrealistic for today's functioning level. The guidelines for quantifying the current level of care and mental status are important in accurate assessment and in helping the client move to a more protected and supportive environment (Conger & Moore, 1984).

Close interaction with the patient is time consuming for professionals. Yet, is is known from the literature that as the patient's age advances, the time of the provider–patient encounter decreases. Considering predictions that in a few short years almost 60 percent of all patients will be elderly, demanding 75 percent of the provider's time, it is imperative that a means of extending needed services in the most efficient manner be found (Lamy, 1982b). An important and necessary distinction must be made between the delivery of medical services and the furnishing of comprehensive health care. Both medical service (or service that makes life possible) and comprehensive health care (or care that makes life worthwhile) directly enhance the self-esteem and functional ability of the chronically ill (Bangerter & Smith, 1981).

References

Bangerter, R. S., & Smith, L. L. (1981). Assessing functional abilities of elderly outpatients. *Health and Social Work, 6,* 40.

Ben-Sira, Z. (1984). Chronic illness, stress and coping. *Social Science in Medicine, 18,* 725–736.

Conger, S. A., & Moore, K. L. (1984). *Social work in the long-term care facility* (reissue). New York: Van Nostrand Reinhold.

Cupit, G. C. (1982). The use of non-prescription analgesics in an older population. *Journal of the American Geriatrics Society, 30* (Suppl.), S76–80.

Gershon, S., & Herman, S. P. (1982). The differential diagnosis of dementia. *Journal of the American Geriatrics Society, 30* (Suppl.), S58–66.

Glenn, M. L. (1982). Family illness rituals. *The Journal of Family Practice, 14,* 950–954.

Greenblatt, D. J., Divoll, M., Abernethy, D. R., & Shader, R. I. (1982). Physiologic changes in old age: Relation to altered drug disposition. *Journal of the American Geriatrics Society, 30* (Suppl.), S6–10.

Grieco, A. L., & Kopel, K. F. (1983). Self-help and self-care in chronic illness. *Southern Medical Journal, 76,* 1128–1131.

Lamy, P. P. (1982a). Over-the-counter medication: The drug interactions we overlook. *Journal of the American Geriatrics Society, 30* (Suppl.), S69–75.

Lamy, P. P. (1982b). Therapeutics and an older population: A pharmacist's perspective. *Journal of the American Geriatrics Society, 30* (Suppl.), S3–5.

Lamy, P. P. (1986). The elderly and drug interactions. *Journal of the American Geriatrics Society, 34,* 586–591.

May, F. E., Stewart, R. B., & Leighton, E. C. (1977). Drug interactions and multiple drug administration. *Clinical Pharmacology Therapy, 22,* 322–328.

Mayo, L. (1956). Problems and challenge. In *Guides to action on chronic illness* (pp. 9–13, 35, 55). New York: National Health Council.

McGlone, F. B. (1982). Therapeutics and an older population: A physician's perspective. *Journal of the American Geriatrics Society, 30* (Suppl.), 1–2.

Rose, J. C. (Ed.). (1985). Nonprescription drugs and drug interactions. *American Family Physician, 31,* 97–98.

Scharlach, A., & Frenzel, C. (1986). An evaluation of institution-based respite care. *The Gerontologist, 26,* 77.

Schilling, R. F., II, & Schilling, R. F. (1987). Social work and medicine: Shared interests. *Social Work, 32,* 230–234.

Sloan, R. W. (1983). Drug interactions. *American Family Physician, 27,* 229–239.

Strauss, A. L., & Glaser, B. G. (1975). *Chronic illness and the quality of life.* Saint Louis, MO: C. V. Mosby.

Viney, L. L., & Westbrook, M. T. (1981). Psychological reactions to chronic illness-related disability as a function of its severity and type. *Journal of Psychosomatic Research, 25,* 513–523.

Williams, M. E., & Hadler, N. M. (1983). Sounding board: The illness as the focus of geriatric medicine. *New England Journal of Medicine, 303,* 1357–1360.

EXPANDING THE ROLE OF FAMILIES OF THE MENTALLY ILL

Marilyn Kaffie Rosenson, Agnes Marie Kasten, and Mary Elizabeth Kennedy

Working with unprepared families is one of the great challenges of deinstitutionalization. The revolving hospital door, the mentally ill homeless, and untreated mental patients in the criminal justice system are problems in the community because of the lack of adequate support services for discharged patients. As these enormous cracks become more visible, social workers need to examine the potential for expanding the role of the family.

It has been estimated that up to one third of chronically mentally ill persons, and as many as 65 percent of all individuals discharged from inpatient psychiatric facilities, return to the family home or nearby, thereby requiring the family as a major source of support (Goldman, 1982). How can we help these relatives avoid the burnout that comes from chronicity and repeated intermittent crises? What is the best way to bring families to an understanding of mental illness that may facilitate a therapeutic milieu and prevent disappointment in the patient when response is slow in coming? How do we involve the family as part of the team and encourage their long-term commitment? What can be done to engage the family as part of the mental health system, to teach them to become enlightened consumers themselves, and to guide them in planning for their relative's future? Finally, what kind of role can family leaders play in developing a more comprehensive mental health delivery system?

The issues and elements involved in expanding the role of families are explored in this article on three different levels: (1) the individual family unit, (2) the group, and (3) the system. On each level the goal is to mobilize the strengths of family members to deal with an extreme life situation in the most productive way.

The Family

How can we help relatives avoid the burnout that comes with chronicity and repeated intermittent crises? On the one hand, there is the necessity for skills used in crises. On the other hand, the skills required to live with chronicity are as demanding, but different.

The most important message a social worker can convey to family members is that while they did not cause the illness, there is reason to hope they can take steps to make a difference in the patient's rehabilitation. Herein lies the significance of the National Institute of Mental Health studies of psychoeducational approaches that equip families with information and problem-solving skills and permit a patient on minimal medication to remain out of the hospital. Christine Mcgill, a social worker with the team of Boyd and Falloon, oversees this four-pronged study, confirming the recent observations of researchers attempting to meet the needs of families with a seriously mentally ill member (Goleman, 1986).

Surveys of families portray a great deal of dissatisfaction with their past experiences with mental health professionals. Families that were left to fend for themselves felt abandoned (Holden & Lewine, 1982). In a recent article, Iodice and Wodarski (1987) refer to the "dumping" on ill-prepared familes and the severely limited access to aftercare programs that have led to much frustration and despair. They recommend the psychoeducational model, which usually incorporates an educational approach within a group setting.

Families need the kind of support that reaffirms their value. In general, professionals are finding that traditional family therapy is counterproductive for biologically based afflictions such as schizophrenia, bipolar disorders, autism, and Alzheimer's disease (Johnson, 1986). On the other hand, when the practitioner offers supportive family counseling or acts as a consultant, both the family and patient benefit.

Supportive family counseling is analogous to support one may offer to the family of a patient with a serious and chronic medical illness. Such an illness can exact a severe emotional and financial toll, taxing the family members' ability to cope and demanding a redefinition of their roles and expectations. Bernheim and Lehman (1985) found that "the patient's illness has profound effects on the family, and the family's responses to the patient can have a major impact on the patient's subsequent adjustment" (p. 170).

Bernheim (1982) also noted the family's needs:

> Interventions which ignore the family's needs have the same predictable outcome: they increase the family's level of anxiety, guilt, depression, anger and frustration, and they lower the level of adaptive responding of those people on whom the patient may most need to rely. Instead of alienating the family through avoidance, passive–aggressiveness, or guilt-induction, supportive family counseling tries to develop a therapeutic alliance with family members . . . not only securing the family's cooperation, but repairing their self-esteem and relieving feelings of helplessness which may be seriously reducing their energy stores. (p. 636)

Another successful approach is described by Kanter (1985). A social worker who is now on the faculty of the Washington School of Psychiatry, Kanter served for 10 years as the director of a psychosocial center for chronic mental patients. He finds that successful consultation requires a continual flow of information regarding patient response to the family milieu. The consultant assists relatives in noticing and understanding previously overlooked aspects of patient behavior. They work together to discover, through trial and error, the degree of support and structure at each point in time that will optimally facilitate patient development. The consultant anticipates crises, stressing the preventive value of prompt intervention.

Empathy is the foundation for those methods. Kanter believes that a family consultant should have a background of direct experience with patients in milieu settings, such as halfway houses and rehabilitation centers, in order to appreciate the stresses in the home. Families experience a major upheaval. They face an extreme life situation that causes bewilderment and anguish along with loss and grief. And there is the ongoing worry about what will happen next. Observers have related the experience to the *Damocles syndrome*—like the king with a sword dangling over his head, many live in constant dread.

Dealing with an indefinite stressor is especially wearing. Here, the social worker requires an understanding of the wearing-out factor and compassion fatigue attending a long-term illness that has no forseeable end. Women in particular experience the feeling of being trapped into giving up their life goals indefinitely, and deinstitutionalization has been called a "women's issue" in that it disproportionately affects the lives and welfare of women (Thurer, 1983).

Empathy comes from listening actively as family members tell what this catastrophe is like for them and for others affected. Empathy grows out of an appreciation of the open wound and the need for healing that may never be complete because it is so enmeshed with unfinished grief. Bernheim and Lehman (1985) expand upon supportive family counseling.

> Through supporting ventilation of feelings, dispelling erroneous expectations, attending to the content of family members' communications, allowing them to set the agenda, refusing to dodge or deflect questions, and adopting a relaxed pace and attitude, we hope to undo some of the iatrogenic effects which may have occurred in the past and develop a sense of mutual trust and cooperation. (p. 62)

In short, empathy is derived when one human being reaches out to another and extends the guidance so desperately sought. The social worker can assist families by explaining the available and state-of-the-art options.

The kind of help that members of a family are ready to receive depends largely on where they are in the phases of adaptation. As with any major upheaval, illness, or loss, there are stages that individuals experience in coming to terms with mental illness (Terkelsen, 1987). Here, difficulties are compounded by the stigma that society and the media promote and by widespread myths about mental illness. Typically, the earliest reaction is one of denial, and the illness is explained by the trials of adolescence, or perhaps street drugs, with the likelihood that the patient will snap out of it. This response is a natural and predictable one, and the worker has to be careful to respect the struggle and to adjust expectations accordingly. Besides, the hope that the patient will pull out of this first episode and lead a normal life is still a realistic one, because for almost 30 percent of all cases, it actually happens (Torrey, 1983).

For those who do have subsequent episodes, families need to be prepared for long-term involvement. Among the first things a family needs to know is that individuals suffering from serious mental illness are considered to be inherently more vulnerable to stress. As the natural link to the community and the world, relatives can be prepared by clinicians to assist the patient in adjusting to the inevitable stresses of transition from hospital to society.

In equipping a family to take on this role, the social worker focuses on meeting the family's need for understanding the illness and treatment options, for practical management and problem-solving techniques, and for knowledge about available community resources. The goal is to promote the coping skills for providing a predictable, low-stress environment with realistic expectations.

It is when the family acquires an understanding of what it is dealing with that a balance can be achieved between the need for support and the need for autonomy. With self-assurance, the fears that provoke overprotection and overinvolvement can be allayed, and relatives are more willing to set necessary limits, demand acceptable behavior, and encourage the patient to take on responsibilities. To do this effectively, the family must learn to accept gradualism as the key and to recognize that sometimes step-by-step improvement can include a step backward. Also, the family will need help in planning for the future when the ill member may be ready to live in the community. Ultimately, relatives must plan for the day when parents can no longer offer the major source of support.

To prepare families, some psychiatric centers have developed short-term family education programs for sharing information. Atwood and Williams (1978) found that the opportunity to meet with other families helped remove the sense of isolation. Another method is used by the director of social services at Southeast Louisiana Hospital—she leads an ongoing open-ended family meeting weekly at the hospital and an additional weekly discussion group in New Orleans for families who have difficulty traveling or whose ill member has been discharged.

Connecting with the family at the time of hospitalization can lead to cooperative discharge planning, which fits in well with the team approach. The use of multiple disciplines has become standard for psychiatric facilities. In keeping with the biopsychosocial view of mental illness, a multidimensional model that incorporates the rehabilitative and educational model is supplanting a unilateral medical model with good results. The acceptance by relatives of the patient as part of the team fits into the overall framework: their understanding of the treatment can be a strong influence on whether or not their relative uses it as prescribed.

One way of involving the family in the team approach takes the form of comonitoring the early signs of decompensation. Throughout this process, the consultant, the patient, and the family meet together to develop an objective list of changes for which to watch (Lukoff, Liberman, & Nuechterlein, 1986). Individualizing and narrowing the number of changes to watch for gives family members a feeling that they have a part in, as well as some control over, what happens. Relatives become adept at recognizing when to contact the professional who can work with them to lower their stress level and adjust the patient's medication, if necessary. The professional's prompt attention conveys the importance of immediacy of response to avoid rehospitalization and promotes the family's willingness to be caretaker.

For families in the caretaking role, setting limits becomes especially important. Sometimes still floridly psychotic patients are discharged and return to the family home where they must be provided the equivalent of 24-hour hospital care. To meet the human need for respite from a round-the-clock job that in the hospital was handled by three shifts, family caregivers need permission to find a way to give themselves a break. When the ill member becomes stronger, relatives can be encouraged to resume activities that enrich their lives with something to look forward to on the calendar. Some may have to put the illness in perspective and avoid an exaggerated sense of responsibility that is nonproductive.

To accomplish this balance, a client may be referred to a day program or psychosocial rehabilitation center. Once familiar with the options, the family can assist the client in accessing community services and in applying for disability entitlements. The curtailment of government funds has had a profound effect on the availability of services, particularly in the oil patch, where state budgets have been hard hit. In some instances in New Orleans, for example, families are performing many of the tasks of case managers. "Well-trained" families can be helpful in linking the client to essential resources.

Intagliata, Willer, and Egri (1980) suggest that a systematic study be conducted to identify those complementary aspects of case management responsibilities that may be beneficial for willing family members to assume.

Being able to play this kind of active role has significant psychological benefits for families. Doing something about a problem helps in dealing with anger and frustration. It overcomes the sense of powerlessness and the potential for depression that can undermine a person's adaptive capacities. Furthermore, as advocates and links to the private sector—including business and civic organizations, churches, private agencies, and associations—family members represent a constituency that cuts across the population. Now that the option of joining hands with other families and working together in groups is available, those who are most familiar with the shortcomings of the mental health system can be motivated to press for change.

The Group

How do social workers involve the family as caretakers and encourage a long-term commitment to the patient? Evidence is mounting that awareness of the benefits of the group process can be fruitful. Approximately one-half million self-help groups dealing with just about every aspect of life have sprung up around the country. Recognizing the group's potential role in prevention, social workers

---

have initiated, facilitated, and made referrals to mutual help organizations (Toseland & Hacker, 1986).

Sharing experiences with others helps families of the mentally ill realize they are not alone. This form of self-destigmatization encourages the move "out of the closet" for relatives from all walks of life, including psychiatrists and social workers. Torrey (1983), whose sister suffered from schizophrenia, believes that the single biggest advance in coping with mental illness since the introduction of antipsychotic drugs is the advent of family support groups.

Some agencies have chosen supportive family group counseling, a professionally led method that teaches specific skills for reducing stress. The instruction is enhanced by the exchanging of ideas and by the understanding family members offer each other. Furthermore, as seen by Atwood and Williams (1978), "groups appear to foster a rapport between family members and the staff that is reflected in how a family as a whole, including the patient, responds to the patient's treatment program" (p. 422). Often a professionally led group stimulates families to form an autonomous self-help organization, and many practitioners view this development as a self-perpetuating vehicle for help with the continuing problems of mental illness and disability.

Educational approaches to families take the form of classes, survival skills workshops, or formal group counseling. Dr. Carol Anderson and her colleagues in the Department of Psychiatry at the University of Pittsburgh have developed a successful family management program that offers education and support while emphasizing a low-key environment (Goleman, 1986). Other centers offer their own version of family support and education, and several clearly written family manuals and instructor's guides are proving to be useful tools (Hill & Balk, 1987). In general, agencies working with families who must cope with serious mental illness find that a group setting contributes significantly to success.

Atwood and Williams (1978) found that family group counseling helped the relatives and also benefited the patients. Positive behavioral and attitudinal ramifications resulted from the ventilation of negative emotions that free psychic energy; the grief work that shifts away from loss to what can be gained through building on the handicapped person's remaining assets; reducing guilt, which relieves the psychological pressure to overprotect and infantilize; the sense of safety in the group that promotes self-acceptance and a willingness to make changes (p. 421).

Mental health workers are finding that making referrals to support groups is an effective approach to helping families. Because members of self-help groups often use professional social services more wisely, the group can serve as one component of a multimodal approach for expanding the role of families. Such groups do not depend on government funding and can survive even in times of severe fiscal restraints. As a method of healing, the groups cost little and give their members a chance to provide help as well as receive it. Emphasizing natural networks and the growth of competence, professional social workers can facilitate by providing material support such as a meeting place; serving in public relations and linkage functions by connecting traditional services, clients, and self-help groups to one another; serving as consultants to self-help groups by speaking at meetings, providing training, or providing information about community resources; and beginning self-help groups (Toseland, Palmer-Ganes, & Chapman, 1986).

To initiate family support groups in New Orleans, planners used an educational series designed to meet family's needs (Hatfield, 1978). The subjects covered meeting the family's need for factual information about the illness, medication, and its side effects; for understanding the illness; for coping strategies and management techniques; and for knowledge about community resources and how to access them. Relatives were encouraged to continue with their own lives, balancing the needs of family members with the needs of the recovering relative. After five weeks of meeting with other family members and discussing common problems, many participants were ready to continue. Interested persons were divided into five family support groups by zip code in April 1982. Three more groups, including one especially for people dealing with bipolar disorders, were added later.

While there are common characteristics, no strict model is followed. Each has adopted a path of its own in response to members' needs. The open policy of welcoming families wherever and as often as they wish benefits people whose needs vary over time.

A New Orleans family, dealing with a son who was destructive of property and kept them constantly intimidated because of his large size, sought help from a family group. Although some members had extensive experience with their own situations and the problems of others, none was enduring such extreme conditions, almost a caricature of what can go wrong in a family home when deinstitutionalization goes awry. In fact, some observers conjectured that it was Dr. Raymond Swan's experience with this family in private practice that inspired his study of National Alliance for the Mentally Ill (NAMI) families at the Tulane University Wisner Family Research Center. The questionnaire for his study was piloted among New Orleans family groups (Swan & Lavitt, 1986).

It took a long time for this particular family to change conditions in their home. They continued to live in constant dread, even though members of the group were supportive and explained options. Finally, after attending the support group meetings for 18 months, they took action and called the police. When their son had been hospitalized for a few weeks, he told them he understood their situation and did not blame them. Today he is living in a community apartment program and visits his family; he even cooked his mother a dinner for Mother's Day.

Now, as experienced members of the group, these parents have gained the confidence to provide input and feedback to others, an important part of the self-help process. Some theorists believe that perhaps the greatest healing mechanism is being able to assist others. Kurtz and Powell (1984a) report that "Classic therapies relate to the sufferer only as recipient, thus perpetuating the self-concept of weakness and failure" (p. 15). Here "one is not only good enough to receive help but to give it as well" (Kurtz & Powell, 1984, p. 15). It is a self-affirming interdependence that encourages competence. The helper therapy principle posits that people in the helper role gain in self-esteem and cognitive experience. Those who help reap benefits for themselves—sometimes even more than the people they help. They seem better able to cope with their own problems as they help others to remedy theirs.

Thus, the mechanisms of mutual help are specifically useful to families of the mentally ill and the self-help group can be viewed as a complement to professional services. Here is a way for families to acquire both the skills needed to deal with recurring crises and the equally important but distinct skills needed to deal with chronicity. To handle intermittent crises, the family requires the assurance of ongoing access to a mental-health consultant, who, with empathy, can help them learn to watch for certain signs, to plan ahead, and to receive an emergency response. And for the long haul, for the years of living with a chronic long-term illness, the group offers support and everyday management techniques. Observing the growth in competence when families learn to work together to regain stability in their lives has encouraged an increasing number of social workers to use self-help groups as community resources.

In turn, groups welcome referrals from social workers and often bring in mental health professionals as consultants. Several of the New Orleans groups invite a mental health professional every month to discuss a specific topic with their members. The benefit of these kinds of programs has been described by Lefley (1983) who related what one woman said after a year of meeting with a family support group in Miami:

> During the last year I have heard psychiatrists talk about mental illness and psychotropic medications; social workers on dealing with

crisis situations and how to handle the demands of living with a mentally ill person; and lawyers and judges on disability payments and on estate planning to make sure our loved ones are taken care of when we are gone. And many other things like these. I have had 14 years of experience with hospitals and mental health professionals, but no one told me any of these things. Last year at this time I was still alone with my problem and totally overwhelmed. CAMI [Community Alliance for the Mentally Ill, Miami, FL] has given me security. Now I have some answers to some questions, and if I don't have the answers, I know other people who do. (p. 1)

As social workers and other professionals are invited by group leaders to share information and exchange ideas with members at meetings, a process occurs that makes for positive relating. Through interaction, families and practitioners develop mutual respect, concern, and understanding at a time when severe budget limitations make such a relationship a practical necessity.

Thus, the group provides a pathway to eliminate the practice of excluding families and to overcome the obstacles to building an alliance for the benefit of the patient. Clinicians are beginning to encourage families to provide information that is tremendously important to the treatment team. Relatives know a lot about prodromal signs and the patient's earlier response to specific medications. The concerns about confidentiality are waning as professionals recognize that the kind of information the family seeks regarding treatment, expectations, and management does not intrude on the privacy of the patient. Additionally, it has been observed by Bernheim (1987) that most patients during a stable phase are willing to sign a consent form to share information with their families.

> If the family brings the patient to the hospital for admission, they are obviously aware of the patient's hospitalized status and at least some of the factors contributing to it. In fact, their input may be critical to decisions regarding hospitalization and immediate clinical interventions. There is no breach of the patient's confidentiality if someone on the treatment team talks to them about their perceptions and knowledge about the patient's illness and problems. (Bernheim & Lehman, 1985, pp. 60, 61)

Groups are important for expanding the role of families by breaking down barriers between families and mental health professionals. Dissatisfaction with the mental health delivery system and treatment by mental health professionals can be ameliorated. It is the blaming stance on the part of practitioners as perceived by families that has done the most to alienate and undermine the alliance. The group offers an avenue for overcoming this major barrier.

Professionals, in meetings with the family groups, are taking the opportunity to clarify matters regarding biomedical causal factors in schizophrenia and depressive and manic-depressive disorders. This can make a substantial difference in the way relatives relate to clinicians. A good illustration of how this happens is seen in support groups for the families of victims of Alzheimer's disease. In this illness, caretakers are becoming more involved and assertive as they are informed of the biological factors (Teusink & Mahler, 1984).

A professional who subtly, or not so subtly, blames family members will undermine their ability to adapt and can jeopardize the bond. Most social workers now recognize this and welcome approaches that seek to mobilize the strengths of families for the benefit of their clients (Arieti, 1979). However, as always, there is resistance on the part of some individuals. It is therefore recommended that if, after reviewing the current literature and attending major professional conferences, a worker remains uncomfortable about relating to families in this educational and supportive way, another area of specialization should be considered. Too much is at stake here: for every turned-off family, there is the potential for another homeless mental patient.

Within the groups, families are learning that they have choices. According to the Group for the Advancement of Psychiatry (1986), practitioners who are locked into old theories of causation and pathology fail to understand the kind of information they need. Local family groups share with each other advice about which professionals their members have found to be supportive and which ones they have not (Eckholm, 1987). Regardless of the setting—hospital, agency, or private practice—families seek out professionals whom they feel are able to understand their problems.

For practitioners in private practice, working with family groups has also been instructive in another way. Within the framework of the group, family members are able to articulate concerns about restrictive insurance coverage and the extensive financial burden that psychiatric treatment entails. The heavy drain on the family coffers becomes a great strain for a middle-class family with other dependents. Eventually, chronic mental illness takes too great a toll. By accommodating a treatment plan to personal budget constraints and by bringing in other resources, the consultant enables a patient and the family to continue to use private help that otherwise could become prohibitive.

Mental health administrators are beginning to appreciate more fully the impact of the immense gap in availability between private and public hospital beds. Psychotic persons voluntarily seeking relief and asylum, unless considered dangerous, are frequently put back on the streets because of the shortage of public beds. They are "seen but not admitted (SBNA)," and have served as the subject of studies under that category (McRae, 1983). Nowhere is the distinction between haves and have-nots greater than in the availability of inpatient psychiatric services: voluntary patients who are able to pay are not likely to be SBNA at private facilities. Instead, such hospitals are advertising for them on television.

It is these shortfalls in the mental health delivery system that groups should be encouraged to address in their advocacy efforts. A family movement of enlightened consumers can press for much needed changes.

The System

"What's good for consumers is good for the system." Building upon this premise, Congress has mandated that those most affected by the mental health delivery system have an advisory role in planning and monitoring services (Peters & Lichtman, 1979). Families and direct consumers participate on advisory and governing boards of mental health centers, planning councils and committees, protection and advocacy projects, group home monitoring programs, state legislative task forces, advocacy coalitions, and advisory committees.

The role of families as activists is changing the way professionals and family members relate to each other. Legislative advocacy is an important function that families are learning to fulfill, often with the guidance of mental health administrators. Numbers mean political clout when lawmakers are contacted on behalf of the mentally ill. Administrative officials, who are employed by the state, are prevented from entering the political arena, so the effectiveness of the citizens' group is valued. Issues such as defeating proposed funding cuts for community programs, and laws affecting insurance coverage for psychiatric treatment are often dealt with by family groups.

When public mental health clinics in New Orleans were on the chopping block, a citizens' campaign of letters to legislators and newspapers averted what could have been an incalculable loss. The Greater New Orleans Mental Health Coalition is composed of representatives from mental health center advisory boards and leading mental health organizations who have banded together to advocate with the Louisana Legislature. One method used is the issuing of legislative alerts through a telephone tree of family members who call or write their respective lawmakers.

Families can be encouraged to contribute to the system in other ways. They need to be cognizant of the value of family support linking community services to other parts of the system. Families who help patients access services and other resources play a central role in making the system work as intended. If a resource that could be appropriate for the mentally ill goes underused, it may dry up or change direction. Therefore, it is important to make the family and family groups aware of what is available. Hatfield (1985), a leading authority on mental health issues involving families, reminds us that families are consumers too:

> Those services we use tend to stay in business while those we avoid tend to drop out. There is potential consumer power in the decisions we make. Informed consumers may do more to promote the effective services and weed out the ineffective than professional standards and peer review can ever hope to do. (p. 1)

In some places, expanding the family's role in accessing services for the patient has gone still further. In a regional developmental disabilities service system in California, for example, family members are trained to assume case management responsibilities. As reported by Intagliata, Willer, and Egri (1986), "in this program, interested family members attend a formal training course and may eventually work as their relative's certified case manager under professional supervision. While we are not advocating that families of the mentally ill become so integrally involved with their relative's treatment, the success of this pilot program demonstrates the desire and capability of many family members to carry out important case management functions" (p. 706).

For the community support system to fulfill its promise, collaboration with families in using community resources is a major step forward. Among the 10 essential community support system functions described by Judy Turner, three are particularly useful for this discussion: (1) backup support to families, friends, and community members; (2) involvement of concerned community members in planning and offering housing or working opportunities; and (3) case management to ensure continous availability of appropriate forms of assistance. The original NIMH report noted that 11 major federal agencies and at least 135 programs were relevant to the needs of CMI persons. The systems approach has been designed to involve these resources for community survival (Turner & Tenhoor, 1978).

Expanding on this awareness, a family group in Pittsburgh, sparked by a grant to a mental health agency, developed a resource and information booklet used by the entire mental health community. Many professionals now see the value of sharing information with families, and this is useful in reducing the long wasteful period of trial and error to find the best approach for a given patient.

The family, as an entree to the private sector, offers another method for developing resources. A church or civic organization can be brought into service by providing a site and/or funding for special programs. Churches offer shelter and meal plans and meeting rooms. Families can be encouraged to influence church programs on a broader basis and seek out knowledgeable clergy sensitive to the needs of the mentally ill who can influence their peers.

When it comes to funding services, providers and families are natural allies. In deciding to refer families to self-help groups, Bernheim and Lehman (1985) observe that professionals may need to overcome their own resistance. Sometimes it is necessary to look beyond an uneasiness about the potential for initial tension in order to reap the benefits. The self-help group's capacity to counter helplessness, defeatism, isolation, and loneliness more than compensates for whatever tension is provoked between consumer and professional" (p. 167). The authors find that advocacy activities result in greater self-esteem, a sense of accomplishment, and diminution of helplessness. They recommend that clinicians educate families about the opportunities available for advocacy and about ways to begin to get involved.

Administrators can inspire a group with possibilities and opportunities for sparking or initiating badly needed programs. Some family members have the need to see concrete results from their efforts, such as a psychosocial center or group home. This has been observed particularly with men who are accustomed in their businesses or professions to adopting a "take charge" stance. A child's mental illness can bring a great deal of frustration and the loss of the sense of control may be overwhelming. Social workers can guide such relatives to work constructively. They can join the efforts described by Starr (1980) of "families who used their ingenuity, energy, and dedication to convert their despair and personal tragedies into innovative programs which run the spectrum from drop-in centers and 24-hour crisis lines to independent residences, sibling support groups, anti-stigma efforts, writing and sponsoring legislation, and altering state health insurance practices."

In a study of the role of family groups in fostering community support programs, Levine (1984) reported on 36 NAMI affiliates located throughout the country. Services ranged from Waterville, Maine, where an apartment serves two people at a time, to Queens Village, New York, where hundreds of members are involved. Usually, they consist of residential quarters with support, drop-in centers, or psychosocial rehabilitation facilities that offer vocational training and transitional employment. The study was performed four years ago and many more groups have since become involved.

The Friendship Club in New Orleans was formed this way. A psychosocial rehabilitation center now serving more than 200 chronically mentally ill persons, the Friendship Club was developed by families with the guidance and encouragement of Louisiana administrative officials who served as catalysts. Wise officials and effective family leaders worked together and learned from each other as they developed a full-time comprehensive facility governed entirely by a lay board of families, friends, and patients.

The Friendship Club is the product of an ongoing collaboration with family members in the community support movement. Encouraging families to go beyond the role of shaping the therapeutic milieu for the patient in their midst by reaching out to change the system can be good for the family's mental health as well as for the system. Researchers who have studied service programs in state mental health systems find that the best programs are closely tied to active family groups. Torrey (1983) says that it is no coincidence that the strongest state AMI groups are found in the states ranking highest in services for the mentally ill, because this represents a cooperative effort.

An interesting extension of family influence on quality of care are the programs for monitoring community residences. The process involves trained volunteers who visit group homes for chronically mentally ill persons to observe and report on conditions. Many of the volunteer monitors are relatives of someone who has a severe mental illness, and they are particularly sensitive to the problems of community living.

Enlightened self-interest is a strong motivating force, and the more family members understand about how limited the options are, the more involved they can become. The goal of autonomous community living for an individual patient can be achieved when there are appropriate resources for housing, vocational, and social opportunities. These supports are necessary for survival and may continue to be necessary. For this reason, families in some areas of the country have began to seek guidance in planning for the day when they are no longer around, and social workers need to know how to help. As reported in the AMI Newsletter (Staff, 1987):

> This fall joint effort was initiated with the Association for Retarded Citizens (ARC) to establish two statewide organizations to aid us in caring for our mentally ill dependents when we are either unable to do so or are no longer here to do so. The two organizations being planned are a pooled monetary trust and a surrogate parent program . . . we hope ultimately to include other similar groups in the trust and the surrogate parent program . . . . The Wisconsin Community Trust for the Disabled . . . will permit individual trusts to be pooled and managed as a single trust but still retain their individual

identity . . . . The Surrogate Parent Program would attempt after your death to substitute in some degree for the personal care and oversight of your dependent that you now provide . . . the surrogate program would only supplement, not replace, existing support programs and provide care oversight and advocacy. (p. 2)

Similar programs are being considered in other states. Virginia has Planned Lifetime Assistance Network (PLAN), which has reached the stage where trained staff can advise families about living arrangements, health care, job placement, recreation, and monitoring of services and medication outside the hospital.

As federal funds are curtailed, the importance of the reassurance these programs provide is growing. Agencies whose policy it is to make referrals to support groups are finding it to be a cost-effective way to help the family cope. In some instances, professionals and family members are forming partnerships to compensate for shortcomings and advocate for change. Making sure that advisory and governing boards retain a substantial percentage of family members and consumers as mandated by Congress is a procedure that does not entail more dollars.

Professionals are mobilizing the strengths of individuals who represent a broad spectrum of expertise by encouraging family members to take an active part in using and developing community resources. Because mental illness affects all economic and educational groups, including doctors, lawyers, businessmen, and even social workers, there is a pool of talent to offer support. Mental health administrators and concerned families are discovering that they share mutual concerns and interests, and enlightened families are becoming effective allies.

References

Arieti, S. (1979). *Understanding and helping the schizophrenic: A guide for families and friends.* New York: Simon & Schuster.

Atwood, N., & Williams, M. E. D. (1978). Group support for families of the mentally ill. *Schizophrenia Bulletin, 4,* 415–425.

Bernheim, K. F. (1982). Supportive family counseling. *Schizophrenia Bulletin, 8,* 636.

Bernheim, K. F. (1987, February). *Key parameters in programs for families.* Paper presented at the NAMI Conference on Educational Approaches to Families, Washington, DC.

Bernheim, K. F., & Lehman, A. F. (1985). *Working with families of the mentally ill.* New York: W. W. Norton.

Eckholm, E. (1987, March 17). Schizophrenia's victims include strained families. *New York Times,* p. 1.

Goldman, H. H. (1982). Mental illness and family burden: A public health perpective. *Hospital and Community Psychiatry, 33,* 557–559.

Goleman, D. (1986, March 19). Aid in day-to-day life seen as hope for schizophrenics. *New York Times,* p. B12.

Group for the Advancement of Psychiatry, Committee on Psychiatry and the Community. (1986). *A family affair, helping families cope with mental illness: A guide for the professions.* New York: Brunner/Mazel.

Hatfield, A. B. (1978). Psychological costs of schizophrenia to the family. *Social Work, 23,* 355–359.

Hatfield, A. B. (1985). *Consumer guide to mental health services.* Arlington, VA: National Alliance for the Mentally Ill.

Hill, D., & Balk, D. (1987). The effect of an education program for families of the chronically mentally ill on stress and anxiety. *Journal of Psychosocial Rehabilitation, 10,* 25–40.

Holden, D. F., & Lewine, R. J. (1982). How families evaluate mental health professionals, resources, and effects of illness. Schizophrenia Bulletin, 8, 626–633.

Intagliata, J., Willer, B., & Egri, G. (1986). Role of the family in case management of the mentally ill. *Schizophrenia Bulletin, 12,* 699–708.

Iodice, J. D., & Wodarski, J. S. (1987). Aftercare treatment for schizophrenics living at home. *Social Work, 32,* 122–128.

Johnson, H. C. (1986). Emerging concerns in family therapy. *Social Work, 31,* 299–306.

Kanter, J. S. (1985). Consulting with families of the chronic mentally ill. In *Clinucal Issues in Treating the Chronic Mentally Ill* (New Directions for Mental Health Services, #27). San Francisco: Jossey-Bass.

Kurtz, L. F., & Powell, J. (1984, May/June). *How do self-help groups work?* Paper presented at the National Council on Community Mental Health Centers Annual Meeting, New Orleans, LA.

Lefley, H. P. (1983, May). *Community support: An alliance of clients, clinicians, and caregivers.* Paper presented at the Region VI Conference on Community Support System, New Orleans, LA.

Levine, I. S. (1984). *Developing community support service programs: A resource manual for family groups.* Boston: Boston University Center for Rehabilitiation Research and Training in Mental Health.

Lukoff, D., Liberman, R. P., & Nuechterlein, K. H. (1986). Symptom monitoring in the rehabilitation of schizophrenic patients. *Schizophrenia Bulletin, 12,* 579.

McRae, J. (1983). Seen but not admitted at the state hospital. *Psychococial Rehabilitation Journal, 7,* 21–32.

Peters, S., & Lichtman, S. A. (1979). *Citizen roles in community mental health center evaluation: A guide for citizens.* Rockville, MD: National Institute of Mental Health.

Starr, S. (1980, August). President's address at the Annual Meeting of NAMI, Chicago, IL.

Swan, R. W., & Lavitt, M. R. (1986). *Patterns of adjustment to violence in* families of the mentally ill. New Orleans: Elizabeth Wisner Research Center, Tulane School of Social Work.

Terkelsen, K. (1987, February). *The family consultation: A new role.* NAMI Conference on Educational Approaches to Families, Washington, DC.

Teusink, J. P., & Mahler, S. (1984). Helping families cope with Alzheimer's disease. *Hospital and Community Psychiatry, 35,* 152–153.

Thurer, S. L. (1983). Deinstitutionalization and women: Where the buck stops. *Hospital and Community Psychiatry, 34,* 1162–1163.

Torrey, E. F. (1983). *Surviving schizophrenia: A family manual.* New York: Harper & Row.

Torrey, E. F., & Wolfe, S. M. (1986). *Care of the seriously mentally ill: A rating of state programs.* Washington, DC: Public Citizen Health Research Group.

Toseland, R. W., & Hacker, L. (1986). Social workers' use of self-help groups as a resource for clients. *Social Work, 30,* 232–237.

Toseland, R. W., Palmer-Ganeles, J., & Chapman, D. (1986). Teamwork in psychiatric settings. *Social Work, 31,* 46–52.

Turner, J. C., & Tenhoor, W. J. (1978). The NIMH community support program: Pilot approach to a needed social reform. *Schizophrenia Bulletin, 4,* 319–344.

Staff. (1987, May). Organization Report, *Wisconsin AMI Newsletter.*

CONTRIBUTORS

Editors

John S. McNeil, DSW, is Professor and Director of The Community Service Clinic, Graduate School of Social Work, The University of Texas at Arlington.

Stanley E. Weinstein, PhD, is Chief of Social Work Services for Mental Hygiene, and Director of Manpower Management, Maryland Department of Health and Mental Health.

Authors

Joan P. Bowker, PhD, is Director, Shelter Management Training Project at the Henry Street Settlement, New York City. From 1983 to 1987, she served as Director, Council on Social Work Education Curriculum and Resource Development Project on Chronic Mental Illness. She recently edited the book *Services for the Chronically Mentally Ill: New Approaches for Mental Health Professionals.*

Shirley A. Conger, MSW, is a consultant for nursing homes and hospitals in the metropolitan Los Angeles area. She also is Instructor, Graduate School of Gerontology, California State University at Fullerton and at Chaffey Community College. She has published several papers and coauthored the book *Social Work in the Long-term Care Facility.* She serves as Secretary to the Long-Term Care Council, California Chapter of NASW.

Laura F. Davis, PhD, is Chair, Department of Social Work, University of Wyoming, Laramie. She served as Curriculum Development Specialist for the American Public Welfare Association in Washington, D.C. She contributed to the book *Services for the Chronically Mentally Ill: New Approaches for Mental Health Professionals,* published by the Council on Social Work Education in 1988.

O. William Farley, PhD, is Professor, Graduate School of Social Work, University of Utah, Salt Lake City. He is Past President of the Utah Chapter of NASW.

Mark Fraser, PhD, is Director, Social Research Institute, and Associate Professor, Graduate School of Social Work, University of Utah, Salt Lake City.

Donald K. Granvold, PhD, is Associate Professor, Graduate School of Social Work, The University of Texas at Arlington.

Kenneth A. Griffiths, EdD, is Professor, Graduate School of Social Work, University of Utah, Salt Lake City.

Agnes B. Hatfield, PhD, is Professor Emeritus of Education in the Department of Human Development, University of Maryland, College Park. She serves as Coordinator of curriculum and training for the National Alliance for the Mentally Ill, Arlington, Virginia, and as Director of Family Education, Maryland Department of Mental Hygiene in Baltimore. Her book *Families of the Mentally Ill: Coping and Adaptation* was published in 1987.

Audreye E. Johnson, PhD, is Associate Professor, School of Social Work, University of North Carolina, Chapel Hill.

Lou Ann B. Jorgensen, DSW, is Acting Associate Dean and Associate Professor, Graduate School of Social Work, University of Utah, Salt Lake City. She is Past President of the Utah Chapter of NASW.

Agnes Marie Kasten, MLS, is Leader, Manic–Depressive Support Group, New Orleans.

Mary Elizabeth Kennedy, MSW, is Regional Director of Community Services, Region I, Louisiana Office of Mental Health, New Orleans.

Terry Mizrahi, PhD, is Professor, School of Social Work, Hunter College of The City University of New York. She is Chair, New York City Chapter of the NASW Task Force on Prospective Payment Systems, and a member of the NASW Health/Mental Health Commission.

Kay D. Moore, MSW, is Director of Social Services at Beverly Hospital in Montebello, California. She is a member of the Society of Hospital Social Work Directors, the American Hospital Association, and the Long-Term Care Council of NASW. She coauthored the book *Social Work in the Long-term Care Facility,* and has presented workshops and papers on this subject.

Marilyn Kaffie Rosenson, MSW, is Community Liaison for the Friends Alliance for the Mentally Ill, New Orleans. She also works with the Curriculum and Training Social Work Group of the National Alliance for the Mentally Ill.

Brenda Wiewel, MSW, is Clinical Director of the Los Angeles Centers for Alcohol and Drug Abuse. She is Treasurer and Past Chairperson, Women's Council, California Chapter of NASW.